Anesthesia Conversations

Corey Scher

Anesthesia Conversations

A Novel Perspective to Teaching

Springer

Corey Scher
New York, USA

ISBN 978-3-032-05353-4 ISBN 978-3-032-05354-1 (eBook)
https://doi.org/10.1007/978-3-032-05354-1

This Springer imprint is published by the registered company Springer Nature Switzerland AG
The registered company address is: Gewerbestrasse 11, 6330 Cham, Switzerland

Preface

The evolution of education in anesthesiology has shifted from reading textbooks to question banks and anecdotal clinical experiences. The primary educational goal for residents in training is to just "pass the boards" and for those who have the goal of remaining current, question banks serve them as well. Reading a textbook can be laborious and time consuming but offer a comprehensive approach to anesthesiology. I was and remain a text book reader. The modern day students of anesthesia have joined the ranks of those in the epidemic of shortened attention spells. I am adding to the preexisting literature a book that is inclusive for those of becoming boarded and for those seeking currency. It is a highly unusual book of anesthesia case reports.

Yao and Artusio's *Anesthesiology: Problem-Oriented Patient Management* will always be the model of problem-solving case reports. The first edition was published in 1983. The present version is the 9th edition, which is a testimony for its educational success. *Anesthesia Conversations: A Novel Perspective to Teaching* is also a book of case reports but the cases are embedded in fiction. Is the book a novel? Not quite. Does it match the science of the Yao and Artusio's book? Not quite.

The 56 challenging anesthesia cases include fictional anesthesiologists in fictional settings. The format is designed for the reader to increase the memory of some of the basic fundamentals of clinical management. I did have a case of Alpha-1-Antitrypsin Deficiency years ago. I hope that the appearance of "Kevin McBride" will help you remember the topic and enjoy Kevin's challenges in his life. We all know a "Chris Landry" and "Hesh Green." Chris is the Chair and Hesh is the regional expert." Lily is the program director.

All of the fictional characters practice at Trinity Hospital, which is a homage to the legendary Charity Hospital in New Orleans. Tulane University Medical Center and Charity-LSU will always have a soft spot in my heart. They built the foundation of my academic teaching endeavor. I have been asked about the time line of the book. The cases are post August 29, 2005, the day Katrina hit and thereafter. Healthcare during and around Katrina is best documented by Sheri Fink's *Five Days at Memorial* and Spike Lee's documentary ,*When the Levees Broke: A Requiem in Four Acts*. The culture of New Orleans is authentic and memorable to those who have come to New Orleans for just a weekend or for their lives permanently.

Our lives are nothing more than the addition and subtraction of all of the conversations that we have over a lifespan. Susan Scott's *Fierce Conversations* emphasizes the importance of conversations in shaping relationships, work and life. These conversations make the characters in each authentic.

New York, USA Corey Scher

Contents

Trinity Hospital

1

Trinity Hospital and the Trinity School of Medicine were founded on May 10, 1924, by a grant from Joe E. Brown and his wife, who were known as the most philanthropic people in New Orleans. The clinical mission of the Browns' was to provide elite and comprehensive care for the indigent people with no regard to the patient's lack of resources. The educational mission was to educate students and residents to learn and provide the concept of patient-centered care. The Browns were able to establish a business model for ongoing financing through government allocations, managed through legislative appropriations, local taxes, and private contributions. They formed a group of "Founders" to develop the philosophy for the School of Medicine.

The hospital had various locations over the years, and the most recent version of the 20-million-dollar building is on Tulane Avenue. The Trinity that exists today is an Art Deco 30-floor steel-framed structure faced with dolomitic limestone. The building has a reinforced concrete foundation and is W-shaped with two, 20-story wings. Courtyards between the wings provided natural light and ventilation. The second floor has a psychiatric lockdown unit, and the third floor was believed to be haunted, a rumor that persists to this day.

The wings were separate and were equal but were separate facilities for white and African American patients. This was in accordance with Louisiana segregation laws. Indigent patients line the walls of the waiting rooms, hoping to spend the night under a roof. When care is free, the costs to the city put the public hospital deeper in debt than the year before. The money to provide a standard of care to the indigent was exorbitant compared to other hospitals in Orleans Parish. Trinity had historically been one of the largest public hospitals in the United States with 2680 beds. The hospital was always threatened by the possibility of the loss of federal and state government funding. This did not dissuade the employees from moving forward elsewhere. The goal is to be a "lifer."

In 1932, the Governor of Louisiana, Huey Pierce expanded the Trinity School of Medicine to include every field in modern medicine that had residents and medical students in training. It was envisioned by the Founders of Trinity that recruitment of

C. Scher, *Anesthesia Conversations*,
https://doi.org/10.1007/978-3-032-05354-1_1

students and residents was opened exclusively to residents of Louisiana. It was a must that the Curricula Vitae of applicants included their home addresses and the high schools they attended in the State of Louisiana.

The modern Trinity (1532 Tulane Avenue) while open to students from all states remains the "Mecca" for Louisiana natives. Physicians on the faculty now come from the United States and 20 different countries. The chair of every department in the School of Medicine is from Louisiana, and that will never change. Presently, the Trinity School of Medicine receives more applications than any other medical school in the United States.

The present version of Trinity has 50 operating rooms, 2 operating amphitheaters, 10 anesthetizing areas in the obstetric unit, 1 in the radiology department where interventional procedures are performed, and an operating room in the legendary Trinity Trauma Room (TTR). Just prior to Hurricane Katrina, there were 22 operating rooms.

The TTR is the center of the emergency department's care for violent crime. A squeegee is needed after every gunshot and stabbing, to push the blood away from each trauma slot to get ready for the next round of patients. The TTR room has its own operating room and a dedicated CT scan that runs 24/7. Transporting critical patients adds risk to outcomes. There is no need to transport patients in the TTR. A second operating room is now complete and is ready for "prime time."

The City of New Orleans has annually one of the highest violent crime rates in the United States. The TTR is always full. The trauma program trained hundreds of nurses and physicians to take care of some of the most challenging patients in the country. What is easy to explain, it was rare to leave Trinity despite its limited resources to pay their workers. Cases that are bizarre in all of the New Orleans's metro are simply common at Trinity. A blind man with a gunshot wound is nothing but a humdrum.

The majority of the physicians who work in the TTR are from Louisiana and never stay far from Trinity despite the low pay and challenging working conditions. When a physician or nurse applies for a position at another institution, a resume that includes time in the TTR is a guarantee of acceptance. Time spent there is nothing short of earning a medal of honor.

On August 29, 2005, Hurricane Katrina almost ended Trinity Hospital, a part of the heartbeat of the City of New Orleans. The employees worked tirelessly to keep even the sickest patients alive. Every employee that volunteered to remain at Trinity faced the loss of power, severe heat, lack of refrigeration, anarchy, a minimum food supply, and toilets that backed up. When the 17th Street Canal levee broke, Trinity sustained severe flood damage with the power grid in the basement of the hospital. As chronicled in Sheri Fink's "Five Days at Memorial," the disaster plan at Memorial did not include flooding with evacuation. Trinity did include flooding, but the plan was overwhelmed by a category 3 hurricane. The evacuation of patients from the flooded hospital made national headlines, where patients had to be rescued out through high floodwaters and then be picked up by helicopter.

The citizens of New Orleans, from different and distinct generations, gathered together to arrange funding from local, state, and federal agencies to rebuild the

City of New Orleans and Trinity Hospital. The resilience of the people of New Orleans has a long history of combating hurricanes in a city that is below sea level. The city is kept alive by an elaborate infrastructure of levees, pumping stations, canals, and "neutral grounds" to mitagate the loss of life and property.

One-quarter of the population of New Orleans returned by 2 months after the storm, and one half returned by the fourteenth month. Very few returned after the fourteenth month. A significant number of physicians left New Orleans due to the severe damage to their hospitals. The doctors were left with a lack of necessities to take care of patients. It was calculated by physicians that rebuilding the infrastructure, recruiting nurses, physician assistants, office managers, and, above all, regaining patients would take years. Hundreds of healthcare employees left.

It has been over 20 years since the storm, and healthcare is vibrant again. A new generation of physicians has migrated to New Orleans to be part of the rebuilding process. "Conversations is historical fiction of the rebirth of an anesthesia department with anesthesiologists whose humanism and dignity eclipsed the events in their personal lives."

Suggested Reading

1. Hoover EL. Charity Hospital: from the beginning to either a new beginning or the end. J Natl Med Assoc. 2007;99(5):578–9. PMID: 17534018.
2. Stockinger ZT, Holloway VL, McSwain NE Jr, Thomas D, Fontenot C, Hunt JP, Mederos E, Hewitt RL. New Orleans Charity Hospital—your trauma center at work. J La State Med Soc. 2004;156(3):138–9. PMID: 15233385.

2 Blunt Trauma

Chris Landry, Lily Xuan, Billy Wagner, Laura Garland

A 56-year-old UPS delivery man was leaving a drop-off location and was hit by a drunk driver who lost control and pinned him against the wall of a building. A New Orleans Fire Department ambulance arrived minutes later, and the fire man with number 10 on his helmet extricated the man with the "Jaws of Life."

Fireman number 12 called the newly deployed blood transfusion vehicle and gave directions to the trauma site. The two firemen slid a spine board underneath the patient, and the neck was immobilized with a cervical collar. The oxygen facemask was set at 8 liters. After three attempts, an 18-gauge intravenous catheter was secured in the left antecubital fossa. A second IV was a 22-gauge, placed on the dorsum of the right hand.

The blood transfusion truck had the red cross insignia on both doors. The team on the transfusion vehicle, set up a transportable blood warmer and transfused 2 units of O-negative blood through the 18-gauge IV. Two intravenous units of AB+ FFP (the universal blood type for FFP) were transfused without high pressures through the 22-gauge. Essential fibrinogen from cryoprecipitate and platelets were transfused in the field. Both do not need a blood type.

Chris strolled into the Trinity Trauma Room (TTR) as the Emergency Medical Technition (EMTs) were wheeling the patient on the gurney. The patient had a name: Curtis Washington. Curtis was transferred to a stretcher, screaming in pain, and then became unresponsive. His vitals were better than expected; BP 75/40, HR 120, RR 25, SpO2 100%.

"The first priority is an intubation. Then you can do your thing". Chris was always in charge of the entire emergency room when he was there. The emergency room resident asked if he could do the intubation. Chris knew the resident well. "Of course." A rapid sequence induction with 12 mg of etomidate and 100 mg of succinylcholine was uneventful. Chris did not think that cricoid pressure did anything, but he never said no to it.

The patient went directly to the TTR for a CT scan. The anesthesia care team had a full setup that was changed every day. The trauma team radiologist needed

C. Scher, *Anesthesia Conversations*,
https://doi.org/10.1007/978-3-032-05354-1_2

1 minute to make a diagnosis from the images from the scan: open pelvic fractures and bilateral open femur fractures. The neck, skull, airway, abdominal organs, and thorax were cleared.

The nurses transported Curtis and settled him on the TTR operating room bed. The patient was stripped naked. Blood poured out of the open pelvis. The chief of trauma surgery used an ultrasound probe for a 1 minute exam of the patient's heart. There was no pericardial fluid, and the overall gestaut was that the heart was essentially empty.

Lily activated the Massive Transfusion Protocol. She poured into the reservoir of the rapid infuser, 3 units of PRBC and 3 units of FFP. Chris started an infusion of Leave them Dead (norepinephrine) at 15 mcg per minute. The vital signs, despite the volume and pressure, declined; BP 60/40 Pulse 140, Sat 92. They could not keep up with the hemorrhage.

Lily was in her comfort zone. "The hematocrit of PRBCs is 70 and the Hematocrit of FFP is 0". The hematocrit of blood you are giving has a hematocrit of 35. She assigned two residents on the call team to check blood PRBCs and FFP. There is never enough cryo and platelets in trauma cases. Get them!

We need 1 gram of TXA (tranexamic acid). The majority of surgeons and anesthesiologists believe that TXA stops bleeding. That is totally incorrect. TXA is a fibrinolytic inhibitor. It brings stability to the clot so it does not break down. To be effective it has to be given early. It should have been given in the field first. There is very little fibrinogen in blood. In this patient who is hemorrhaging, Cryoprecipitate should be given as soon as it is available. We need lines!"

Chris was in charge of the overall supervision and coordination of the trauma anesthesiologists. The patient was prepped and draped moments after Curtis arrived in the operating room. There was no way to put in lines with sterility when the drapes are already contaminated. Chris did not care if there was a break in sterility. The norm was to utilize ultrasound to visualize the internal jugular and carotid arteries. The days of using landmarks were over. An introducer in the carotid artery often requires an operation.

The protocol for lines was to secure an arterial line first. Lily went old school and palpated the radial artery. Her stick blew up the right radial artery. She was successful with the opposite radial artery. There was no room for ultrasound guidance to determine the location of the right internal jugular vein and right carotid artery. The left side of the neck had thoracic duct which made it a second choice.

After decades of using landmarks, Leon Wagner found the right internal jugular vein with a 22-gauge finder needle. He then slid a 20-gauge Angiocath that was attached to a syringe on top of the finder needle. While drawing back on the syringe, the syringe filled with dark blood. The syringe was disconnected from the 20-gauge Angiocath, and a wire was passed through the Angiocath. An introducer was passed over the wire. From Leon's experience, he was sure that the introducer was in the internal jugular vein.

It is always assumed that the neck was not officially cleared. The collar was removed, and the neck was turned ever so slightly for cannulation. With ultrasound guidance, it was easy to see the echo dense wire that was inserted into the right IJ. The procedure for "neck lines" included placing two wires into the right side of the neck. The short wire is the one that is in the introducer kit. The long wire is for a triple lumen central line. The brown port of the triple lumen is 16 gauge, and the white and blue ports are 18 gauge. The triple lumen is dedicated to all drugs administered. The "Intro" is for volume. The left neck can be secured in the same manner if it is deemed necessary.

Laura's specialty was point of care tests. On the table behind the anesthesia machine were a Thromboelastogram, stat INR, platelet function analyzer, stat PTT, and glucometer. ABGs were done every 15 minutes with massive hemorrhage. The tests of clotting were not helpful if the bleeding is just surgical. An infusion of norepinephrine was started after the lines were secured. Chris added vasopressin and propofol at 25 mcg/kg/minute. If there was a free port, Chris liked remifentanil at a dose that the patient tolerated.

With lines secured and pressors running, a TEE was inserted to guide volume administration. If there is an esophageal injury, viewing pulse pressure variation is adequate in the completely supine position with the table flat.

Lauren assigned a medical student to draw blood off the arterial line for ABG analysis every 15 minutes. Lauren did not want "gases" drawn, if the TEE revealed an "empty" heart. She waited until more blood products were administered. The ABG after 8 units of PRBCs and 8 units of FFP, with norepinephrine and vasopressin running, was: pH 7.13 CO 52, HcT 22, calcium 6.2 mg/deciliter, potassium 6.7 mEq/L, O_2 sat 92, and a lactate of 8. They were still behind.

One gram of calcium was administered. The reservoir on the rapid infuser was never full. The PRBC/FFP ratio was now 2:1. The ventilator respiratory rate was increased to 15 breaths/minute. The FiO2 was increased to 100%, and the PEEP was increased to 10 from 8 mm/hg. The hyperkalemia was addressed with an infusion of glucose and insulin, terbutaline, and another bristojet of calcium chloride. The new changes in the respiratory rate would hopefully be additive to the other therapeutics.

The surgeons were struggling to isolate bilateral iliac arteries and one vein. The vena cava was not bleeding. The chief trauma surgery suggested packing the pelvis and transporting the patient to interventional radiology for an angiogram to find all of the bleeders.

Lily was now very concerned. The blood bank needed more time to assemble another MTP box. Lily needed a "bridge to transfusion." She had two options. Albumin as a colloid will stay intravascular and support blood pressure if enough is given. Curtis's urine output was only 50 cc since the operation started. Albumin could "clog up" renal glomeruli and contribute to acute renal failure. 5% Hypertonic saline as opposed to 0.9% normal saline will stay intravascular. The oncotic load of 5% saline will be intravascular for 30 minutes to 1 hour. With the pelvis packed, Lily felt less concerned as hypertonic saline seemed to keep the blood pressure up. The transport to interventional radiology was without incident.

The interventional radiologist formulated a plan. The vena cava was intact. The right iliac artery and both iliac veins were the major sources of bleeding. There were numerous small vessels that were bleeding, but they would resolve with time. There was no way out of clamping the right iliac artery and both iliac veins. The patient would die if they were not clamped or embolized. Curtis would surely lose his leg to save his life. Clamping the left iliac vein could result in gangrene. There was no way out to give Curtis a quality of life. There were no Hail Marys in this case.

Lily had the residents transport the rapid infuser to interventional radiology. She transfused unit after unit and knew that she could only catch up with the clamping and embolization of the right iliac artery and both iliac veins. The pressor requirement had not changed. Curtis was transported back to the OR for the surgeons to "mop up" and close. Laura ran another ABG.

pH 7.3. CO2 38 O2 72, Hct 28, Calcium 8, Potassium 7.0! Lactate 10.

"We are running out of time if we do not get the potassium down. Glucose-insulin, terbutaline or any other therapy will take too long. I have a plan that I have read about but have never done." Chris always thought outside the box.

"I need someone to go over to the blood bank and bring me two empty blood bags that have citrate, phosphate and dextrose in them" Chris disconnected the rapid infuser line from the introducer. He opened the line of the introducer and attached a 60 cc syringe. "We are going to draw 60cc of blood out of the patient and infuse normal saline through another line. After 200 ccs of blood is drawn off, we will check an ABG."

Chris told the surgeons to hold off until the hyperkalemia problem was resolved. After 500 ccs of withdrawn blood and 2 liters of saline infused, Laura ran an ABG. The potassium was now 5.4. Lily started to clap, "Brillant."

The remaining threat was Curtis's oxygen level. Chris did an intraoperative bronchoscopy. It was normal. In Chris's mind, the relative hypoxia and all of the FFP administered could in synchrony cause TRALI (transfusion-related lung injury) TRALI made the case even more tenuous. The treatment is supportive, which means that there are no specific treatments.

While the surgeons started too close, there was no visible clot in the surgical field. Hypofibrinogenemia generated by severe hemorrhage was the culprit. At the end of the coagulation cascade is fibrinogen. Lily wanted to administer fibrinogen concentrates, which costs $1500 per bottle. Lily knew that multiple bags of cryoprecipitate would easily exceed the costs of fibrinogen concentrates. The surgeons wanted to know why fibrinogen concentrates are not routinely given.. Lily claimed that it just became available at Trinity.

"I have also ordered PCC; Prothrombin Complex Concentrate. PCC is a blood product that contains factors 2,7,9, and 10. There is no doubt that after this hemorrhage, we are still factors behind."

This is a case where the surgeons often leave the abdomen open. They thought that Curtis was not going to live, so they closed. Chris and the Chief of Surgery stepped out to speak to the family. When they left the OR, the right leg was cold and blue, and the left leg was seemingly ok. Chris spoke first and summarized the steps of the case, from the OR to interventional radiology and back to the operating room. Chris volunteered to bring the family up to speed.

"We did everything possible for Curtis. His right leg needs an amputation and the left leg is likely to develop gangrene. It is hard to say over time what will happen to his left leg. We are going to transfer Curtis to the Surgical Intensive care unit. He will be on a ventilator with infusions of medication that keep his blood pressure up. We are now in the watch and wait mode so why don't you go home and get some rest. It is now ten o'clock. Come back in the morning around 8 AM. From that point on, we will need you to make a plan for Curtis."

The family arrived at 8 AM. The critical care team proposed the plan for the day. The cold, blue right leg required an above knee amputation. Gangrene started in the left leg. The need for the fasciotomy was discussed. The left leg now became a threat to Curtis's life.

The case was more than urgent, and surgery started before the family arrived. The family was devastated. Both legs were amputated under general anesthesia.

"My father has been delivering mail for over 30 years. Walking is his passion. As a bilateral amputee, he will never be able to recover in his mind. This is the worst case scenario. This is not over! This is a fatal injury if not physically but certainly mentally."

Chris's heart was breaking. "At the end of surgery, we made him comfortable with large doses of narcotics."

"He is now on narcotic infusion."

"Does he still need the drugs to keep his blood pressure up."

"He does and the dose of each one has doubled. We did notice a small area of gangrene in what is called the perineum. It is the space between the anus and genitals The infection is called Fournier's gangrene. We will take him back to the operating room at noon to debride it. Debridement means to cut out the infected tissue. We will debride the tissue until we find uninfected borders."

The family could not process all that was going on. Chris knew that Curtis could not be saved. Chris tried to give a message to the family that was clear. The patient suffered a fatal injury, and there was nothing that reversed the process.

At the midpoint of the debridement, the surgeons stopped. The infection was now in the rectum, and there was not enough tissue to cover the area of debridement. The open space was packed and covered with a wound vac. The wound vac was there just to cover the area of surgery.

"Your father is dying. The infection has spread to his vital organs. This infection cannot be controlled. All we can do is make him comfortable. In the old days we used the terminology of "withdrawing care". We will now, with your consent, we will provide comfort care. The first step is to examine him to make sure he is receiving medications for adequate pain relief and sleep."

"Everything that makes a patient seemingly uncomfortable is removed. For example, the catheter of his penis is taken out. We will remove the breathing tube, the tube from his nose to his stomach and leave the narcotic infusion on. We will turn the blood pressure drugs off. The combination of the significant amount of narcotics in his blood and the removal of the breathing tube, will make him pass quickly and comfortably. Of course you will take whatever time you need to make a decision. If you want us to do more, we will but it will not change his outcome."

Curtis died 20 minutes after extubation, Chris was unable to calm the family. During the debriefing, Chris and his team critically reviewed the case. It was concluded that everything that could be done was done.

Suggested Reading

1. Downar J, Delaney JW, Hawryluck L, Kenny L. Guidelines for the withdrawal of life-sustaining measures. Intensive Care Med. 2016;42(6):1003–17. https://doi.org/10.1007/s00134-016-4330-7. Epub 2016 Apr 8. PMID: 27059793.
2. Giles RC. The control of bleeding in disarticulation of the hip by ligation of the common iliac. Vein and artery. Ill Med J. 1954. PMID: 13191817. No abstract available.
3. Grottke O, Mallaiah S, Karkouti K, Saner F, Haas TM. Fibrinogen supplementation and its indications. Semin Thromb Hemost. 2020;46(1):38–49. https://doi.org/10.1055/s-0039-1696946. Epub 2019 Oct 1. PMID: 3157454.
4. Jedlik J, Becker BF, Chappell. The endothelial glycocalyx. Crit Care Clin. 2020;36(2):217–32. https://doi.org/10.1016/j.ccc.2019.12.007. Epub 2020 Feb 6. PMID: 32172810 Review.
5. Lier H, Hossfeld B. Massive transfusion in trauma. Curr Opin Anaesthesiol. 2024;37(2):117–24. https://doi.org/10.1097/ACO.0000000000001347. Epub 2024 Jan 19. PMID: 38390985.
6. Meneses E, Boneva D, McKenney M, Elkbuli A. Massive transfusion protocol in adult trauma patients. Am J Emerg Med. 2020;38(12):2661–6. https://doi.org/10.1016/j.ajem.2020.07.041. Epub 2020 Jul 22. PMID: 33071074. Review. The family decided to come back tomorrow with their decision. Curtis died in the night from a car.
7. Zaza M, Meyer DE, Wang YW, George M, Daniels K, Cardenas JC, Cotton BA, Ng W, Jeratrh A, Wasowicz M. Tranexamic acid: a clinical review. Anaesthesiol Intensive Ther. 2015;47(4):339–50. https://doi.org/10.5603/AIT.a2015.0011. Epub 2015 Mar 23. PMID: 25797505.

3 Rebuilding the Department of Anesthesiology at the Trinity School of Medicine

Chris Landry

Hurricane Katrina decimated all but two anesthesiologists of the full-time faculty of The Department of Anesthesiology, Critical Care and Pain Management at Trinity Hospital. It would take 2 years to restore the critical number of 50 attendings to cover Trinity and all of the affiliated sites. There was a rush to keep all of Trinity's residencies afloat. The federal government provides funds for most medical residencies through Medicare, Medicaid, and Veterans Affairs. The cost per resident per year in these governmental residencies is between 38,000 and 150,000 dollars. This included salaries and education costs.

In order to maintain funding and the education of residents in post-Katrina Trinity, the Baylor College of Medicine, University of Texas-Houston, University of Texas Medical Branch in Galveston, and Texas A&M created the South Texas Alliance of Academic Health Center. Although the Alliance was an excellent opportunity for Trinity residents to continue their training, this was not entirely acceptable to many residents. After the trauma of the storm, many residents just wanted to go home, and certainly not to Texas. All of those who left were accepted into the residency of their choice—one located close to home. Every resident who lived in Louisiana continued their training in Texas, only to return home to Louisiana when the time was right.

Over the first 4 months after the storm, the Trinity School of Medicine laid off 250 faculty members including 180 tenured positions. The Department of Anesthesiology was eliminated. Chris and Lily were the only members of the Department of Anesthesiology who stayed. They were not paid. At the sixth month mark after the storm, patients started to fill the open clinics, and a surgery schedule was slowly growing.

Prior to "Katrina," the Department of Anesthesia was composed of 25 full-time faculty members at the Trinity site and 25 affiliated anesthesia faculty members at outside locations. The outside locations completed the ACGME requirements of those rotations not covered at Trinity Hospital. Besides Lily and Chris, 20 of the full-time anesthesiology faculty members left their positions after the storm, never

C. Scher, *Anesthesia Conversations*,
https://doi.org/10.1007/978-3-032-05354-1_3

to return. The challenge was now rebuilding. The Dean of the University started a search for a new chair for the Department of Anesthesiology.

As with all School of Medicine postings, candidates of any race, color, gender, or cultural background were eligible to become the Chairman of the Department of Anesthesia. Privately, the Dean wanted Chris Landry, a die hard, loyal to New Orleans and Trinity. Chris had outstanding organization skills, business acumen, and clinical skills that were "outside the box." Without any academic activities on his CV, it was of no consequence in the post-storm era. Chris did not apply for the position. The Dean just picked him. After 15 minutes of their meeting, Chris accepted the position and the challenges that the Dean presented to him.

There were no patients when Trinity reopened. The Dean had not yet figured out how he was going to pay the newly recruited anesthesiologists. There was a shortage of office space, department administrators, secretaries, call rooms, a pain management clinic, a fully staffed critical care team, and a conference room; as ridiculous as it may sound, there was only one bathroom in the ORs. The residents were returning from Texas, and there was no one to be a Program Director. Chris offered the position to Lily. She evolved to be the "perfect" Program Director, adored by the residents and medical students on rotation.

The model for the faculty that Chris and Lily conceived was that every faculty member at the Trinity had the same salary, 500,000 dollars a year. Participating in the call system was reimbursed with time. Call was entirely voluntary. Call was based on 7 days of night float. Call people that worked 7 PM–7 AM for a week, earned the next week off. Faculty who did a week of night float had no responsibility to the department for the following week. Benefits received were based on those chosen by the faculty. The healthcare benefit was the same for all. Being treated by Trinity and its affiliates, healthcare was comprehensive and free. Meandering outside of the Trinity Health Care System was not covered. The IRA was through TIAA-CREF. Funding of the IRA was through pretax earnings. Children of the faculty could get their college education in the state of Louisiana University with free tuition.

There was a temporary stay for 6 months on all outside conferences, licenses,. professional fees, and ACLS/BCLS. Restoration of these items, while essential, could not be paid for by the Department. There was space for the construction of offices, bathrooms, and call rooms. The pain management site would be at an affiliated outside facility in Metairie. Work would start on them ASAP.

Chris had one true challenge left: salaries. Salaries were tied to a budget approved by the Dean. A salary was based on the collections received from anesthesia services used. With surgery just opening, anesthesia collections to fund a 500,000 dollar salary were months and possibly years away.

For each candidate accepted for a faculty position, it required a 4-month credentialing process to obtain clinical privileges. When up to full speed, a full-time faculty member would earn 10,000 dollars a week He would add faculty over time to allow collections to accumulate. It would take time for surgery to come up to speed. He could match recruitment with the rebirth of the surgery schedule with a team of per diems and CRNAs. They would be placeholders for the faculty as they were added. Chris and Lily agreed to sacrifice their salaries during this hardship. If none of these measures were helpful. Chris volunteered to take out a million dollar loan from his Hibernia account. The Dean rejected the concept of money coming from a faculty member.

Chris was in the mode of "beggars can't be choosy" with the task of assembling a "first class faculty." With the blue tarps that remained on the roofs of many homes in New Orleans, the city was not ready for "prime time." The new post-Katrina levee system took 17 years to complete after the storm. The system included levees, flood walls, canals, and gates. The system is the largest civil works project in the Army Corp of Engineers. It was completed 17 years after the storm.

The horrific heat and humidity lasting from May through October made many visitors wonder if the city of New Orleans was fit for human habitation. While most of the city recovered, several "wards" populated by the poor, remain unchanged since the hurricane. Chris often paid out of pocket to bring potential faculty to experience the status of healthcare, and the well-being of the city. Rather than "sell the city," he always painted a picture of reality. Chris loved New Orleans, and his perspective was part of the equation.

The American Society of Anesthesiology Annual Meeting was in San Francisco and Chris was allowed to have a booth in the main exhibit area. Lily joined him to recruit faculty. They had five candidates who were genuinely interested. Chris and Lily could not miss any opportunity. Lily and Chris agreed to pay for their dinners at Perry's on the Embarcadero. With wine flowing, alcohol could lead to impulsive decisions. Chris wanted them to come by the booth in the morning. No one showed. The goal was to start the Department with seven board-certified anesthesiologists who had done fellowships in the subspecialties in the field. It was a tall order.

When Chris returned to New Orleans, he had a wow moment. He had 32 applicants within 2 weeks after he posted the faculty positions in three different anesthesia journals. He was sure that the applicants lacked a full understanding of what was going on in the city. His plan was to have four distinct Fridays to have groups of eight to visit the medical center and the city. He did not want to sell the city to the candidates. He made a PowerPoint presentation of what life was like now in New Orleans and at Trinity. Chris was the master of injecting humor into precarious situations.

By the end of the month, only eight applicants decided to move forward. Four were from New Orleans, and the remaining four were from Baton Rouge. Out of eight applicants, four were women.

Chris was ecstatic. The eight recruits needed little information. They "get it."

Two of the recruits' families left the city with no plans of returning. The other six were committed to the city and the state. They were lifers to be. It was time, again, to talk to the Dean. Salary, Salary, Salary!

The leadership of Trinity was able to secure funds from the Trinity Endowment.

The Federal government donated a grant of 100 million dollars earmarked for multiple institutions in New Orleans. The salary question was solved.

With Lily and Chris, there were now eight anesthesiologists. The new faculty members were given emergency rights without delay. Trinity offered no-interest loans for housing, education for children of the faculty, and a 20,000-dollar sign on bonus. Chirs's shopping list of all the essential items for a Department to thrive was all addressed. That process took 18 months. The Department of Anesthesiology was molded to meet the model that Lily and Chris created.

Suggested Reading

1. Fink S. Five days at memorial: life and death in a Storm Ravaged Hospital. Crown-an imprint of Random House. https://www.crownpublishing.com. 2013.
2. Fink S. The deadly choices at memorial. Propublica. 2009.
3. Fink S. Rationing medical care: health officials struggle with setting standards. MinnPost. 2009.

4 Chris Landry: The Chair of Anesthesiology, Critical Care, and Pain Management

Friday nights in New Orleans are owned by the prestigious private school, Isadore Newman. The iconic football team was known for the growth and development of the Manning brothers. There is never an open spot in the bleachers for students and alumni to support their team. Chris Landry never missed a game. He never sat on the bleachers. He was under the bleachers smoking weed with his friends. He knew that if he was caught, there would be no repercussions.

Chris grew up in his home on First Street. The home was designated as a historic location. To qualify as a historic location on the National Register, the home met certain criteria in age, integrity, and significance. The house must be at least 50 years old and looks the same as when it was constructed. The Landry family was among the "First Families" in New Orleans.

Chris Landry grew up with the Sunday tradition of a rotation of dinners at Antoines, Commander's the Palace Cafe, Brennans, and Arnauds. Every lunch on Sundays rotated between Galatoires and Mandina's. The Landrys were woven into the traditional culture of New Orleans. His father was the King of the Krewe of Rex in the same year that his mother was the Queen of the Krewe of Iris; the only Krewe that had only women.

Mondays were always red beans and rice, and Fridays were always fish. The Landrys insisted that their housekeeper turned fish into seafood, seafood gumbo, crawfish with corn and potatoes, and Po-boys with fried oysters or shrimp. He favored Crystal over Tabasco and Dixe over any other beer on the planet. Chris learned to cook and prepare drinks that were hard to find outside the city.

Chris's parents were both corporate lawyers of different firms. His father was the attorney for the Police Department, while his mother was the Assistant Attorney for Orleans Parish. His parents could get Chris out of any jam he was in: countless speeding and parking tickets, driving with a failed breathalyzer test, selling pot to his fellow students, and buying liquor when he was fifteen. His parents were "exhausted" raising Chris.

C. Scher, *Anesthesia Conversations*,
https://doi.org/10.1007/978-3-032-05354-1_4

Chris knew that his family was wealthy. Their income was hardly check-to-check. The family inheritance grew with each generation with investments in oil, natural gas, copper, and real estate. Chris's first car was a fully loaded 700 series BMW. Whenever he asked for something of material value, his parents never said no.

The Louisiana State University (LSU) opened its doors on January 2, 1860. The first Landry that attended LSU as a student was around 1890. As the tale has it, the first words that Chris uttered was "LSU." There was never a doubt that Chris would attend LSU. With no "college pressure," Bs and Cs were just fine. If you stuck in a couple of Ds on his transcript, Chris was still going to LSU.

Chris drove his new car to LSU for freshman orientation. Sometime or somewhere, in Baton Rouge, Chris did a 180 flip. He made his choices for the first semester classes: Chemistry, Statistics, English 101, and European History from 1900 to 2000. His parents were in a state of shock. Chris was "going for it." These were challenging courses that put him on some track for a career. Based on Chris's total lack of anything related to scholastic achievement, they remained dubious yet hopeful.

Four years later, Chris's GPA including organic chemistry, calculus, and physics was 3.75. He was not going to be another John Belushi. Chris was going to medical school.

Chris's medical career started at the Trinity School of Medicine. In his fourth year, he chose to secure a position in anesthesiology at Trinity outside the match. He had enough connections to outright make the Dean quiver. He grew into a faculty position in pre-Katrina Trinity.

By showing up every day at Trinity, Chris established a career in trauma anesthesia. Emotionally, he barely skimmed the surface. While he was seemingly compassionate and humanistic, all to often he had to fake it. He treated his patients with the highest level of dignity. Then true to his close friends, there were days when he was not. Genuine, some days and not every day. If he was acting, that was fine because the product he delivered on most days was excellent.

His passion was teaching medical students and residents. Chris opened his house once a month for the residents to eat, drink, and just hang. Lunch was always from Acme: chargrilled oysters, seafood gumbo, and the peacemaker po-boy. The Landry liquor cabinet was comprehensive, and Chris hired the family bartender to make Sazeracs or anything desired.

Chris worked hard at keeping some of his demons from being exposed to the world outside of him. He became what he had no aspirations for. He was one of Trinity's most treasured faculty members.

5 Anesthesia for Dead Bowel and the Protest

Joe Lofton

Joe Loften was from Compton Los Angeles, where the coveted educational class was "Street Smarts 101". Most of his friends had a GPA of 4.0 in Street Life. Joe's grade was 0.0. Both of Joe's parents served in Vietnam. His mother was a nurse at a makeshift Trauma Hospital in the United States, and his father was a Navy pilot who spent 20 years in the military. His parents made sure that Joe Junior's grades in Street Life were always near an F. They created Joe Lofton, Super Nerd.

Joe's father was a "hard ass." He was a person who followed rules and regulations meticulously and enforced them without exception. Joe Jr. was trained to work hard in school. There was no alternative. Joe never had a grade less than an A. He did not ever want to see the alternative. Joe Jr. was on a path that made him an outcast nerd which was the worst-case scenario for a kid from Compton. He went to his father for advice.

Although Joe's father had a sparkling Silverado pickup truck, he always took the bus with his son when leaving the neighborhood. Everything was a lesson. When they arrived at Sports Authority, Joe Jr. knew to keep his mouth shut and watch his father in action. The first stop was to look at all of the Air Jordans. Joe picked out the 3/4s and not the full high tops. The colors were the iconic black, red, and white with number 23 on the heels. Joe Jr. was taking baby steps away from nerdom.

The next stop was looking at the glass backboards, and orange rims mounted on an adjustable back stop. The ball was Wilson's, and the jersey was Michael's. Joe Sr. welled up and imagined it all set up on their driveway. The pièce de résistance was a gallon of white paint to mark half of a court.

Joe Jr. had an athletic talent that he and his father did not know existed. Joe Jr. had "game" and tenacity. Watching YouTube hoops was an acceptable alternative to studying Waterloo. Joe Sr. broke most of his rules. Balling was now an urgency, and his academic proclivity was on hold. There was a growing bond between seniors and juniors.

Joe Jr. just made the middle school team. He was the 12th man picked for the 12-man team. By the end of the season, he was getting the minutes he needed to

C. Scher, *Anesthesia Conversations*,
https://doi.org/10.1007/978-3-032-05354-1_5

average 10 points a game. He started the season at 5 feet 10 inches and was 6 feet 1 inch at the end. When the season was over, he weighed 180 pounds up from 168 pounds. There was no off-season for the next 5 years: the weight room, playing in the leagues at the Staples Center, travel teams and finally, the all-district league that required an invitation from the voting coaches in the district. This league was a showcase for college recruiters.

Joe Jr. ended his high school career as one of the most respected students at Centennial. Despite his accomplishments of playing hoops, he never lost his title of being a nerd. He evolved to be the person that his parents wanted him to be.

Joe Jr. chose the path that his father spent so much of his life on. He entered the United States Naval Academy at Annapolis and was accepted to the Uniformed Services University of the Health Sciences for medical school. He entered the Naval Medical Center Portsmouth for his Residency in Anesthesiology. The obligatory 5 years of service were at Bethesda Medical Center.

Chris Landry was a basketball junkie and made his annual trek to Madison Square Garden for the first round triple header in the Big East Tournament. Unknowingly, he made conversation with the person in the next seat. He was seated next to Joe Lofton Jr. Joe junior had the gift of conversation. By halftime, they both went for a beer and divulged that they were both anesthesiologists.

After the second game, Chris offered Joe Jr. dinner at the Porter House Bar and Grill. It was only four subway stops from the Gardens on the C train. After two martinis, Joe made it perfectly clear that he was going to make an attempt to recruit him. By martini number 4, Chris offered Joe Jr. an all-expense trip to Trinity and New Orleans; Joe had no reason not to accept the offer. He asked Chris if he could include his fiancé on the trip. Joe had 2 months left in his obligatory service while his fiancé had a month left of service as an interventional neuroradiologist. Chris answered Joe's request to have his fiancé accompany him on the trip, "Simply perfect."

It was Joe's first night call as an attending, and he was scared shitless. He already had seen it all over the years at Portsmouth, but a new environment is always accompanied by a level of anxiety. He had a team of four residents. Chris said all of the right things to calm down a very obviously nervous newbie. "All the residents are battle tested and I selected these residents to take this call. After one case with them, you will be relaxed."

"Roxy," who was the Chief Resident, was on call to steer Joe in the right direction. At 5:00, while Joe was ordering dinner from "Port of Call," all of the anesthesia beepers went off at once. There was a code in the outpatient urology suite. Roxy, who arrived first, opened up the airway box as she was getting a report from the Urology Chief Resident. She was focused on the patient and was not engaged with the report that the urology team was giving her.

All she saw was a cyanotic, gasping, "little old lady." Roxy had the residents put the patient on the floor from the treatment table, to get maximum intubating conditions. After three failed attempts, Joe took over and intubated the patient with ease after he insisted that the patient be transferred back to a stretcher headed to the operating room.

Joe was pissed "Everybody, shut up please! This is becoming a shit show!! Hydronephrosis yes. Is this the problem? Absolutely not. The attempt was to drain the kidney and she collapsed. This case is not about the kidney! Whatever is going on is in her abdomen. Her chief complaint was abdominal pain. That is why she is here. Let's draw some labs and get a C-T. with IV contrast. She is 84 years old. She does not deserve the bias against the elderly which is growing around the country."

There was not a single resident among the anesthesia and urology residents who thought that Joe was correct. Although this was his first call for him at Trinity, Joe let everyone know that he completed an anesthesia residency and a fellowship in critical care at the Naval Hospital in Portsmouth. His military personality began after high school and evolved over the years to become a leader. His status was lieutenant. In the naval hospital, rank was achieved through time and service, Joe was in charge in the operating room and insisted on being called "Sir" and not Dr. Lofton. Yes sir was formal but Joe wanted it the military way. It showed discipline and rank.

His team placed an arterial line, triple lumen catheter for infusions, and an introducer for a Swan-Ganz catheter for pulmonary artery pressure measurements. While there remains a question of the validity of wedge pressures to measure volume status, there are formulas that correlate systemic vascular resistance with the CVP and mean arterial pressures. SVR = MAP − CVP/CO × 80 has a result in dynes/sec/cm^5. The pulmonary vascular resistance is PVR = mean pulmonary artery pressure − pulmonary capillary wedge pressure/CO. These calculations are used for the rational choice of vasopressors. If the systemic vascular pressure is low and the PVR is high, then phenylephrine is a poor choice. The right heart is at baseline under stress, and adding phenylephrine would make the PVR worse. The right heart is a thin-walled conduit to take blood from the cava and direct it to the lungs.

"There are no vasopressin receptor binding sites in the lung. Utilizing vasopressin in this case where the PVR is already high is an excellent choice, The wedge pressure that is measured can be correlated with the beat to beat variability of the arterial line with respiration. PCWP as a guide, by itself is not a precise measurement of volume."

The CT scan was consistent with a dead bowel with multiple perforations. The ABG revealed severe metabolic acidosis. The lactate was 22. Joe inserted a TEE and revealed global hypokinesis, and an ejection fraction was estimated to be 20%.

A norepinephrine/vasopressin infusion was started through the brown lumen of the triple lumen CVP. Joe wanted to wait for blood typing and cross-matching to be complete. The initial hemoglobin was 10. It was inevitable that a blood transfusion was needed, but it was not yet urgent.

The surgeons ran the bowel with the specific goal of finding the superior mesenteric artery. The bowel was blue and the perforations were "all over the small intestine." "Dead Bowel" was in the distribution of the superior mesenteric artery.

"It is likely that there was an embolus at the insertion of the superior mesenteric artery. Joe, is she in sinus rhythm".

"She has runs of A-fib. There is no mention of it from her time in the clinic. According to EPIC, there are no medications for A-fib. Untreated, she probably has more than runs of A-fib. Let's fill her up with some Plasmalyte. When she looks full on TEE, let's start some Amiodarone. There could be clots everywhere!. I will give a bolus of 10,000 units of Heparin and an infusion with the target of having an ACT of 350." The heparin serves to prevent clots from growing in size.

The surgical team was very impressed by Joe's scope of clinical anesthesia. His anesthesia residents were not yet sold on Lieutenant Joe.

The surgical plan was a significant bowel resection and stent/bypass of the SMA. Joe's plan was to medically control her A-fib, adequate anticoagulation, Fill her up with packed red blood cells and FFP, and treat her congestive heart failure.

"Ok team, Let's start norepinephrine at 10mcg, Lasix 40 mg IVP. Let's change the anesthetic to a TIVA with prop/remi/dex and rocuronium. Sevo is a calcium channel blocker and I do not want to treat chronic congestive heart failure (CHF) with Sevo."

"She is having a stroke in her small intestine. We have to do something ASAP. We cannot wait for hours to revascularize her bowel."

Joe stood his ground. "The damage to her bowel is already done. Let's do a quick angio of her head and then make a decision."

"Joe, a clot retrieval will not help her brain. We cannot stop our bowel resection. We passed the golden hour hours ago. It is not how much we take out, it is how much functional bowel will be left? We cannot stop now looking for and retrieving a clot in the brain."

Joe was agonizing over the right plan. He was starting to gain acceptance from everyone in the room.

"Take care of her abdominal surgery first. That is what is more likely to kill her."

The resection took 2.5 hours. A total of 250 cm of small bowel was left in the patient. It was just on the borderline if she had enough bowel to avoid lifelong TPN. During the entire case, she remained in sinus rhythm but was unstable. During the resection, the anesthesia plan continued to unravel with Joe's ongoing evaluation of the heart with TEE.

"The LV appears to be stunned. Blood from the epicardium was not penetrating to the endocardium. She is in heart failure.. We have to unload her. Increase the Propofol infusion to 125 mcg/kg/minute. Double the Remi. Give it a few minutes. Then, we will increase the dose propofol to 150 mg/per minute. If the heart, on TEE, remains hypokinetic, we will start with milrinone. Please inject 40 mg of Furosemide."

"Sir, urine is pouring out of the Foley. Since the initial dose of furosemide , there are 400 ccs in the bag. I think we should give her a second dose. I think that a liter of urine will clearly represent significant unloading. Another dose. Sir?" The Chief Resident and her call team were clearly in agreement with Joe.

"Yes, another 40 mg of lasix again. Stop all the fluids and let's get another gas!"

The pH was 7.29, O_2 110, CO_2 45, K 4.8, Hct 26%.

Joe was getting the positive feedback he needed. "Her FIO2 is 50%. The formula is 5 times the FiO2 should be the optimal oxygen in the blood. Her oxygen level should be 250. Her 110 demonstrates a huge shunt.

I will do a bronchoscopy to rule out the usual. If I do not find anything, we should get a chest X-ray but start ARDS ventilation now. It has been published that early

Adult Respiratory Distress Syndrom (ARDS) ventilation prevents severe ARDS. The post-ARDS ventilation gas was pH 7.3, CO_2 38, O_2 110. On ECHO, I think the EF is 40%. The airway pressure was 45, on the ventilator, down from 53. With an O_2 at 50%, she should have an O_2 of 250.

"Sir, the heart looks much better!" The surgeons were ecstatic. The Cardiology fellow asked "Since the heart looks better, can we put a balloon pump in?"

Joe was not technically in charge but he was now. We do not know where we stand with ARDS. I think the balloon will unload her which will be very helpful. if her airway pressures go up.

"Let's take ten minutes to put the intra aortic balloon pump in with the precise location". The surgeon's confidence in Joe soared with his successful treatment of Chronic Congestive Heart Failure (CHF). The dead bowel was out so the clock slowed down."

Dr. Patel shaved and prepped the groin. The balloon pump took 8 minutes to insert and set up the settings. The TEE looked normal and the dose of Levo was reduced to 5 mcgs./minute. The TEE image remained "almost normal" and Joe wanted to leave well enough alone.

The surgical plan for the end of the case was to keep the patient open. This was a grossly contaminated case and frequent wash outs would be necessary.

The sedation was turned off and TM was asked several probing questions. There was no response. The neurologists wrote in their consultation that a proper neurological diagnosis was not possible. Post-operative delirium and cognitive function decline were likely. It could take weeks until these issues were sorted out. A C-T angio was ordered and there was no evidence of a stroke.

This 82-year-old powerful woman survived. After months in rehabilitation, she was discharged to home to her family with skilled nursing. TM was saved by Joe Loften's team, excellent surgeons and nurses at all levels. Six months had passed since TMs trauma. Joe Lofton was there to "save the world", which gave him affirmation of his choice for a career in anesthesiology.

It was one of those typical New Orleans summer days; blistering sun and 100% humidity. By 4 PM, the skies would turn black, and were ripe for thunder, lightning and rains like a wicked monsoon. After 45 minutes of downpours, the sun, humidity and blistering heat were back. Joe walked to the mailbox at the end of his driveway. There was a letter from the Commissioner of the State of Louisiana. Joe had no idea what was about to happen.

Joe was named in a malpractice case. Essentially, he was being sued by the dead bowel lady. He grabbed the letter and his temper went from 0 to 10 plus. Joe was apoplectic and fuming at the same time. "I saved her life and she is now suing me!!!!" Joe escalated his temper to rage. He felt genuine betrayal.

Joe jumped into his Toyota Corolla and broke the speed limit on Esplanade Avenue. His name was painted on his parking space in the Trinity garage. His walk became a trot and then a sprint as he entered the Medical Record Office. He found TMs medical record and outright stole it. As he walked back to his car, there were so many emotions firing in his brain all at once. Betrayal was smothering him.

Joe pulled off the face sheet that had her personal information. He copied her address and phone number. TM lived in Gretna, on the west bank of the Mississippi

River. Without any self-restraint, he decided to go to TM's house and have her take his name off the suit.

There was a doorbell, but Joe was in such a state, he pounded on the door and waited just a few seconds before he started pounding again. No response. He waited for 5 minutes and a frail, tiny woman opened the door. He did recognize her as the dead bowel lady. Joe introduced himself with the highest level of hostility. She started to cry and slammed the door in Joe's face. He knocked again knowing that she would not answer the door. It was time to get his "shit together" and go home.

There were many names in the lawsuit and he was sure they too, must have made the trip to Gretna. The following day the phone rang in his office. It was the legal department and they wanted to speak to Joe with great urgency. "Right now!!" They wanted to verify that he made a trip to the plaintiff's house.

"That is the most fucked up thing, you could have done. It is a case of harassment that that could escalate to an assault charge not excluding sexual abuse. As of this moment, you are on an unpaid leave of absence! While you are home and digging deep into your fucked-up mind, you must know what really happened. She dropped the suit against you!"

"Why am I suspended? What I did worked! She understood that I had nothing to do with this circus and dropped me off the suit."

"She dropped you because you frightened her and she thought you would come back! A big black man confronts a petite white woman. You freaked her out!"

Welcome to the South. She did file an assault charge. The way that works, "shit for brains." in an assault charge, she is not suing you. The state of Louisiana is suing you! You cannot win this case and we are not representing you. You will have to hire your own attorney. They will ask you to give 20,000 dollars; 5000 for the judge and 15,000 for the firm. That is the only play in town. Since she dumped you, so will we. We will help you with any of your medical fuck ups but not activities outside the School of Medicine."

Joe was devastated. He took 6 mandated months off for treatment of anger management and the needed time to work with a defense attorney at private practice rates. He found a law student who is supervised by law professor Evan Ellegard at the Tulane School of Law. This was not just another assault case. There were several potential powerful legal issues in the case that disqualified it as a teaching case. The case was for himself and his firm of 50 attorneys.

There was no way that Joe could afford the legal fees for Evan Ellegard. Evan was a regular guest on MSNBC and had spent 20 years as a government prosecutor who specialized in civil rights. This was the kind of case that could wake up any bored or burnt-out attorney. The case was discussed by the partners of the firm at their monthly dinner meeting, and it was unanimous that the case would be free of any fees for Joe.

At least 10 junior attorneys in the firm that were engaged in comprehensive research on TM and her family looking for any history of racism. There were 10 senior attorneys that passed the Louisiana bar, and one was a full partner in the firm, Evan Ellegard. Not one of the attorneys in the firm's Louisiana division thought that Joe had committed a felony or simply violated any law. "It was an understandable temper tantrum."

The "comprehensive" research lasted one whole hour. TM had three sons who joined the Neo-Confederates 10 years ago. The group initially wanted to restore life in the South in the Confederacy Era but have evolved to be, if possible, more extreme and now resemble most Neo-Nazi groups.

"We have contacted the FBI for more information. They track every right wing extreme group with details about all of its members. Their information on its members is comprehensive and we need to know how we can get information. It is likely that the majority of their intel is not for sharing and is for national security."

Evan Ellegard was tenacious. "I will get the information of these three assholes. As a former civil rights attorney, I do not think at all of this information is under lock and key. I have security clearance with the FBI to gather data when it is clear that the data had little to do with our national security."

"I am looking for data that is referred to as "superficial intel". I will have a report ready in five to ten days and will bring Joe up to speed on what we are doing. From time to time, there are clients that do not approve of our game plan. I would be shocked if Joe did not approve of our work. This case will not go past the deposition. TM will drop Joe from the assault charge in one minute or less."

Joe did not believe that a race card was the way to go, but Evan Ellegard showed his experience and wisdom when information from the FBI poured in. TM lived in a world of racism. Her sons had a rap sheet of arrests involving white supremacy. TM did not come to the deposition, and her attorney dropped the charge.

Suggested Reading

1. Piiccirillo M, Graf GJ. Medical malpractice: a case study in medical and legal decision making. Yale J Biol Med. 1989;62(1):23–42. PMID: 2728499.
2. Puch EA, Nowak-Jaroszyk M, Swora-Cwynar E. Medical error in theory and practice - a review of the most important issues. Med Pr. 2020;71(5):613–30. https://doi.org/10.13075/mp.5893.00988. Epub 2020 Sep 15. PMID: 32969411.
3. Ravddin I. Anesthesiologists, surgeons and malpractice suits. Anesthesiology. 1959;20(3):377. https://doi.org/10.1097/00000542-195905000-00018. PMID: 13650224.

The Department of Anesthesia's Residency on Probation

6

Lily Xuan

As Program Director, Lily privately thought that the life and culture of New Orleans made the city a fantastic place to spend a weekend, but not a day more. The city had difficulties attracting Fortune 500 companies to set up shop. The negative perception of New Orleans stemmed from the fact that the city was built below sea level, with a history of hurricanes, violent crimes, and crushing heat and humidity. The poor economy would never change, and dangerous public housing was a topic that no politician wanted to bite into.

The public school system was far from being vibrant. The children of transplanted companies would have an inferior education which led to a "game over" sentiment for companies to come to the "Big Easy." Orleans parish ranks 67th out of 68 school districts in Louisiana. Lily was spot on. New Orleans was a tough sell to out-of-staters.

The path that tourists view includes the French Quarter and several stops along the streetcar track; the Garden District, the "Wedding Cake House," Tulane University, Audubon Park, and onto the Riverbend. Everyone falls in love with the city, but the sentiment changes when they migrate away from the carefully selected streets of the "Crescent City." The claim that too much of the city is not safe is backed by data on violent crime, which is perennially near the top in the country. Everyone on the Trinity faculty can share a story where they were a victim of a crime. Crime is a death sentence for retaining faculty members and recruiting residents. Mardi Gras and the Jazz Fest can only take a city so far.

Prior to Katrina, the Trinity anesthesiology residency was on probation with a history of multiple citations. The citations included sexual harassment, a substandard educational curriculum, poor board scores, resident transfers, and failure to meet the educational objectives of the ACGME. No one is applying to residency on probation in a city that is getting very negative press. She had Chris's support to face a giant uphill battle to restore the residency to a seamless level.

Lily sat in Chris's office, and she had a "definitive foolproof" plan for a total reversal and restoration of the department. The professionalism of faculty and

C. Scher, *Anesthesia Conversations*,
https://doi.org/10.1007/978-3-032-05354-1_6

residency will be restored. Lily had a newly found infectious enthusiasm for the new paradigm of resident education and faculty career development.

"Chris, I want to make the residency program and faculty a department of diversity". This conversation is 100% between us. What I propose cannot be shared with any one, period. We are going to be a residency of diversity in terms of culture, gender and race. Simply stated, Diversity, Equity, and Inclusion. Of course that includes all communities. Resident recruitment is not based on the USMLE exam. It is based opportunity. If the Republicans cringe, we are doing the right thing.

On our new website, there will be a picture of 20 fourth-year medical students: 12 of those students will be of color, and 12 will be women. The students will consent to be part of the picture. I have already passed the idea to the Dean. He approved. We will use social media to show our picture and a statement by me that makes this philosophy clear. ERAS opens up in 2 weeks. We will show a detailed plan on our website that includes our strategy to come off probation.

There will be an initial Zoom interview. I will determine which applicants will come to Trinity for a formal interview based on the Zoom session. We will cover all expenses except transportation. They will stay one night. They will have dinner with the residents and lunch with the faculty. There will be four interviews for each applicant. Unlike any other program in the country, the applicants can bring a significant other.

There were 20 citations that led to probation. Lily worked closely with the ACGME to have a rebirth of the residency.

With consensus from the leadership of the Medical School, Chris simply fired those involved in severely crossing the line of professionalism. Three faculty members involved with sexual abuse/assault were fired. Those victims of the behavior of the three faculty members over the years were asked by the Dean if they wanted to press charges. They did. The Dean offered the group legal counsel. There would be no legal fees. The charges were likely to make it to the media with a potential of added negatives to the School of Medicine. The School of Medicine was willing to take on risk. There are no secrets in NOLA.

Lily presented all of her activities to Chris. He supported every initiative to make the department a desirable place to work for both the faculty and residency. Chris was involved only with the faculty and Lily with the residency.

1. Chris appointed faculty leadership positions in each subspecialty of anesthesia.
2. Each subspeciality leader would develop an educational curriculum with a manual and sentinel papers in their field.
3. Rotations for each subspecialty would only be at Trinity Hospital, except for Pain Management.
4. CRNAs would be hired to "refine the educational experience" of the residents.
5. An Intranet would include contact information of faculty members and residents, links to access the medical school library, required courses such as ACLS, True Learning, and general department announcements. Protected

academic time would be allowed based on the time needed for a research idea and the development of the idea into a clinical investigation.
6. Resident case logs would be sent to Lily every Friday.
7. Same sex call rooms and bathrooms would include cable TV and a desktop computer.
8. Faculty office space and a resident lounge would be available.
9. Journal Clubs would be held monthly and hosted at the home of each faculty member.
10. There would be an one-month elective rotation in London, UK.
11. Call would be voluntary for residents—1 week of night float is followed 1 week off.
12. A development of a research endeavor would include every member of the department.

Lily was successful for each bucket list item and arranged for a stat ACGME inspection. The processes went live in 6 months after the inception of the blueprint to take the residency off probation. ERAS opened two months after the final citation was addressed.

Suggested Reading

1. Nagasaki K, Nishizaki Y, Shinozaki T, Shimizu T, Yamamoto Y, Shikino K, Fukui S, Nishiguchi S, Kurihara M, Katayama K, Kobayashi H, Tokuda Y. Association between prolonged weekly duty hours and self-study time among residents: a cross-sectional study. Postgrad Med J. 2023;99(1176):1080–7. https://doi.org/10.1093/postmj/qgad04.
2. Nasca TJ, Miller R, Brigham TP. The ACGME single accreditation system: alterations in the Force of Graduate Medical Education. Acad Med. 2021;96(8):1097–9. https://doi.org/10.1097/ACM.0000000000004111. Epub 2021 Jul 27. PMID: 33788784.

7 Brianna Ortiz: Director of Research-Owner of a RO1 Grant for Phantom Limb Pain

Brianna Ortiz

The new Dean of the School of Medicine was on a single-minded maniacal path to "renovate" the production of quality clinical research in every department. Chris felt like he was a target, and he was.

Chris arranged a gathering for the entire department to discuss a new academic curriculum. It would take dinner and a full bar to capture attention for clinical research. While Lily was saving the residency, the Dean wanted a research plan for the department. Although the new Dean was invited and present at the gathering, he denied all funding for any party. He held the opinion that all parties, including the graduation of the residents, were not part of the School of Medicine.

Chris could have asked each faculty member to "chip in," but avoided the utter chaos that could break out, by paying for it all. All of the residents and faculty were invited. There were five known researchers from the department of surgery to lay out the process of clinical research, starting with a clinical question to developing a project design. Chris added each researcher to the Grand Rounds Conferences.

Chris arranged the menu for passed food as well as sit-down dinner. Chris's goal was to show the Dean that there was no inertia on the research endeavor. He invited the Dean to sit next to him. The Dean talked Chris's ear off which made Chris order a fourth martini.

In his hungover morning, Chris remembered only a few sentences from the Dean. He did remember his tirade about research. Chris had no experience or interest in research. The Dean gave Chris 48 hours to make a presentation on the development research in the department of anesthesiology. Chris had one drum beating down on his head.

Who is going to pay for the research endeavor? He needed anesthesiologists to bill, not sitting in their offices doing, research that more often than not goes nowhere. To start, he needed one full-time board anesthesiologist, two research assistants, each with a Masters in Clinical Research. The Harvard University School of Medicine offers virtual courses that lead to a Masters.

C. Scher, *Anesthesia Conversations*,
https://doi.org/10.1007/978-3-032-05354-1_7

Chris had a plan; academic productivity would be incentivized. Each academic project was rewarded with time off. He wanted to reward research with cash, but there was no free cash in the department.

Menu for Academic Productivity:

- Any peer-reviewed publication in Anesthesiology or the IARS Journal—1 month off.
- Any peer-reviewed paper that is cited in PubMed—3 weeks
- Chief Editor of an Anesthesia Book or Editor of a Journal—3 weeks
- Chapter Writer—2 weeks
- Presenter at a National Meeting—1 week
- Invited Speaker outside of Louisiana—1 week
- NIH funding—1 month
- Industry Funding—3 weeks
- Teacher of the Year—3 weeks
- ASA or IARS committee member—1 week
- All other academic activities—to be determined

Brianna Ortiz

While Brianna's last name is Ortiz, neither she nor her parents spoke a word of Spanish. The family dates back to the late 1800s. As far as Brianne could tell, they were Dominican. There was no Spanish culture in their lives. Her father and mother homeschooled her until the ninth grade, when they placed her in an elite private boarding school.

Brianna graduated with a B.S. degree from the University of California-Berkeley. She completed her medical school, anesthesia residency, and pain fellowship at the Oregon Health-Science Center. Brianna was one of the few who just "breezed" through her education.

Brianna sent out her CV to all of the academic programs in New Orleans, Jckson Mississippi, and Florida. The Trinity department secretary checked Chris's Trinity email no less than four times a day. She printed the CV that was addressed to Chris. The sender was Brianna Orttiz M.D.

Chris was jubilant after reading Brianna's CV. By year 5 on faculty at Oregon Health Science Center, she amassed 25 peer-reviewed papers, edited 3 books, and had a leadership position on the ASA Committee on Pain. She lectured at 15 medical schools in the United States and 10 in Western Europe. Brianna ran the comprehensive pain fellowship at Oregon.

Chris made a one-hour morning telephone call, and by the end of the day, Briannea Ortiz was set to be interviewed for the new Chief of Pain Management and Chief of Research. Chris invited her and her husband Lee to New Orleans to interview and be driven around the city by a realtor. Their flight landed at 4 PM, and they were sitting at a table for four at Commander's palace by 6 PM. Chris always showed up at a table with a cocktail in hand, signifying that it was "cool" to order a drink without judgment.

Lee was actually the target at this recruitment dinner. Brianna could easily envision her life as a member of the department, but Lee needed Chris to help him find his passion living in New Orleans. Chris was not aware that Lee was from the Big Easy.

Lee and Brianna went to New Orleans for a better life. With an academic low salary income, Brianna moved into a section of the house that Lee grew up in. His parents bought a home in Old Metairie that had four bedrooms and made a separate apartment on the first floor. Lee could not get up a flight of stairs, but he had a drop in his pain score for the moment. He was home.

Brianna's husband, Lee was suffering from an extreme case of phantom limb pain that developed after an explosive device amputated his right leg below the knee while serving in Afghanistan. He was sent to Germany for stabilization and then to Walter Reed to be treated for phantom limb pain (PLP).

Lee's pain was in his right lower leg where it used to be. There was no relief from pregabalin, neurontin, opioids, mirror therapy spinal cord stimulator, transcutaneous stimulator, and NSAIDs. While opioids did work, tolerance and addiction required supervised weaning. Lee remains on suboxone.

The true pathophysiology of this horrific condition had not been fully elucidated. In the periphery, PLP resembles the neuronal changes seen in other neuropathic pain conditions. However, in the central nervous system (CNS), imaging studies suggest changes unique to PLP, such as cortical reorganization.

Brianna was not prone to showing emotions but did not hold back when it came to her husband, Lee. She swore to Lee and to herself that she would discover a therapeutic that was undeniably effective for phantom limb pain (PLP).

Briannea landed an RO1 grant that provided the money for resources needed to investigate gene replacement as a treatment for phantom limb pain. While there were studies on the effectiveness of gene therapy for pain, Brianna was a pioneer in investigating gene replacement specifically for phantom limb pain. There was clearly plenty of room to form a new team that included residents, fellows, and co-attendings

Brianna's pre-funding research was focused on all research involving gene replacement for phantom limb pain. There were reports indicating Dorsal Root Ganglia (DRG) stimulation could be an effective treatment method for phantom limb pain in mice. Brianna's team could not find randomized control trials or observational studies with large sample sizes in humans that allow for adequate power to support her gene replacement approach to PLP treatment for phantom limb pain.

Chris did not understand the details of Brianne's investigation. He needed a "dumbed down" version. Chris had a scheduled meeting with the Dean in 2 days.

"Chris, the goal is to inject new genetic material at the site of an amputation, CSF, or into the Dorsal Root Ganglia (DRG). that results in an increase of GABA receptors. The DRG, are bundles of neurons at most spinal cord levels. The DRG injection requires a laminotomy and a microscopic guided needle for visualization. Gene replacements enter neurons when genes are attached to a vector; typically a virus. The new gene replacement causes the virus to replicate leading to more GABA receptors. GABA is an inhibitory substance which moderates and dampens signals in the periphery and central nervous system. Pain is significantly reduced. Is that clear Chris."

Brianna started her project on rats in a randomized, double-blinded trial. The major findings were that the gene replacement was safe and effective after 1 month. She was able to move on to humans, specifically Lee. Lee met no selection criteria to be in the study. He was not part of randomization and blinding. This was clearly not acceptable according to her RO1 grant. If anyone found out about Brianna's personal research, she could lose her grant and be subjected to disciplinary action, not excluding termination. She would treat Lee after the next phase was completed.

She enrolled 50 patients for an "observational component" looking for safety and efficacy of DRG gene therapy. All PLP patients were healthy. There were no adverse effects in any patient. The gene replacement therapy improved their pain scores by 50%. GABA was clearly a factor.

These results raised more questions concerning the project that were not in the grant. Is there a dose-response relationship? Could a vector carry a new set of genes to express another inhibitory substance? Does the site of the amputation matter? Brianna needed to continue the project to phase 2 that achieves power in the study before moving on to phase 3. As the number of patients increased, the power of the study increased and pain scores changed to an improvement of pain by 60%. Brianna thought that the pain relief of 50–60% was simply too low. All of the previous therapeutics that did not improve Lee's pain relief had a success rate of 50%.

Brianna's research team was disappointed by the study. The study was too broad and did not have cohorts of patients who shared common features. It was time for the main focus of her grant: a randomized double-blinded study of DRG gene replacement in PLP patients who had failed conventional therapies.

After a minute of self-reflection, it was time for Lee to be treated. On a Saturday night, when the lab was closed, Brianna injected the stump of Lee's amputated leg with adenoviral genes. Lee had a 75% reduction of his pain in 2 weeks! Three months after the treatment, Lee was pain free. Mission accomplished. Brianna went back to following the steps of her grant precisely. Her resolve to properly perform the investigation was back. Although Lee's success did not count as data in the study, Brianna was convinced that he did count.

Suggested Reading

1. Campo-Prieto P, Rodríguez-Fuentes G. Effectiveness of mirror therapy in phantom limb pain: a literature review. Neurologia (Engl Ed). 2022;37(8):668–81. https://doi.org/10.1016/j.nrleng.2018.08.005. Epub 2020 Sep 19. PMID: 36195376.
2. Collins KL, Russell HG, Schumacher PJ, Robinson-Freeman KE, O'Conor EC, Gibney KD, Yambem O, Dykes RW, Waters RS, Tsao JW. A review of current theories and treatments for phantom limb pain. J Clin Invest. 2018;128(6):2168–76. https://doi.org/10.1172/JCI94003. Epub 2018 Jun 1. PMID: 29856366.

3. Kaur A, Guan Y. Phantom limb pain: a literature review. Chin J Traumatol. 21(6):366–8. https://doi.org/10.1016/j.cjtee.2018.04.006. Epub 2018 Dec 4. PMID: 30583983. PMCID: PMC6354174.
4. Srinivasan N, Zhou B, Park E. Dorsal root ganglion stimulation for the management of phantom limb pain: a scoping review. Pain Phys. 2022;25(8):E1174–82.

Is Anesthesia Safe? Neurodegeneration in Premature Babies Exposed to Inhaled Anesthetics

8

Samantha Dixon, Sofia Gangliano

Clinical Research starts with a clinical question that needs to be asked. Brianna's question for the first faculty research project was "Is anesthesia safe?" To Brianna, "safe" referred to the possibility of neurodegeneration in neuroplastic children stemming from inhaled anesthetics. If true, could these findings have an impact on cognitive function in their lives? While the literature is replete with trials to solve this question, the clinical question remains at best, controversial.

The project had to have a definite answer; different from most investigations that end in "add to the pre-existing literature" or "further investigations are warranted." Brianna, like all investigators, wanted a firm outcome unlike others.

Sophia Gangliano and Samantha Dixon wanted this project as soon as they opened their email. Brianna gave it a thumbs up for Sofia and Samantha. Samantha was concerned that Sofia was impulsive, stubborn, and unpredictable as like a loose cannon. Sofia was always all over the place. Samantha had her own set of issues. Both were able to focus together on the clinical question at hand.

Brianna gave Samantha and Sofia some background. "It has already been established that beta-amyloid protein, Tau protein and apoptosis were discovered in the central nervous system of mice after breathing sevoflurane. The time of exposure was brief as the lifespan of CNS of a rat is brief. These facts launched countless studies to determine if cognitive function was an endpoint."

The research group, the GAS consortium, compared cognitive function in ex-premature babies who received either neuraxial anesthetic or sevoflurane-induced general anesthesia for hernia repair between birth and 60 weeks post-conceptual age. The infants were assessed at 5 years of age with tasks of attention, memory, sensorimotor development, exploration, concept formation, and problem solving. There was no difference in cognitive test performance at 5 years between the children who received spinal anesthesia and those who received sevoflurane. This investigation was published in Lancet.

This excellent work convinced Brianna; yet, there are significant ongoing investigations to clarify the clinical question. We should take a shot at that. There were

C. Scher, *Anesthesia Conversations*,
https://doi.org/10.1007/978-3-032-05354-1_8

many limitations in the study. New research is ongoing, and there is certainly room for the work of Sofia and Samantha.

"Read the study and go to the most recent studies on PubMed. Try to come up with some thoughts on what is left that has to be investigated. This process is called research or in law 'Discovery'. Brianna, a fan of this study, thought that criticisms needed criticism."

Samantha knew the topic well. "The consortium was years ago. Where are we today? There have been countless papers that have had different results, and the topic remains controversial. The clinical question, hypothesis and project design must be straight forward. I believe that the sample size must be larger than most previous investigations. The sample size must match the project design of a meta-analysis. We will collect data from independent studies on this topic to determine trends. We can then analyze trends to elevate the level of the investigation."

Sofia was not intimidated by Samantha's preexisting knowledge. Sofia had her own level of preexisting knowledge. Sofia took the role of an attending who introduced to the residents and students the topic of neurodegeneration in neuroplastic babies after sevoflurane. She was proud of her passion to follow the literature on the topic. She referred to specific papers and their authors. While Sofia had the reputation of being handicapped by her wild swings in her moods, she was able to focus on this topic. She exposed Samantha to her comprehensive knowledge of the literature on the topic.

A fight rather than an agreement developed. Sofia should have, but did not anticipate Samantha's working knowledge of the clinical question and vice versa. Samantha broke the world record for being aloof that matched Sophia's temper.

Samantha was pissed off. "It is now my turn to show off." "You sound like you were quoting the abstracts. Did you actually read these papers? It doesn't sound like it! In case you did not read the actual study, here it is!"

Since the GAS studies, published in Lancet, there have been over 20 papers from excellent peer review journals that are emphatic that this matter remains unsolved. We need our own clinical question which will evolve from previous studies.

As in Sophia, Samantha was more than familiar with the literature. She cited what she referred to as sentinel papers. She did not summarize the GAS paper. She, for the most part, memorized the Lancet paper. Samantha cited studies after the Gas Consortium paper. Then she referred to papers that were both compelling and were current. Brianna stepped in as a referee.

"Samantha! Sofia! Stop! Stop!

Brianna wanted them to obtain data that would result in an association or better, an experimental design that shows causality. "A case control, pro or retrospective cohort design, and cross-sectional design would take forever to accrue enough patients to substantiate an association. An experimental design, as in double-blind models, is not possible because randomization and parental consent are both difficult to attain and exhausting. As you have said, the best project design for your study is a meta-analysis. You are using preexisting data which is needed for a meta-analysis. A meta-analysis" indicates that the review includes a statistical synthesis of results from at least 2 of the included studies".

Samantha gave a list of papers that would be essential to be included in such a meta-analysis.

1. McCann ME, de Graaff JC, Dorris L, Disma N, Withington D, Bell Morton N, Berde C, Soriano S, Davidson AJ, et al. Neurodevelopmental outcome at 5 years of age after general anaesthesia or awake-regional anaesthesia in infancy (GAS): an international, multicentre, randomised, controlled equivalence trial. GAS Consortium. Lancet. 2019;393(10172):664–77. https://doi.org/10.1016/S0140-6736(18)32485-1. Epub 2019 Feb 14.
2. Wu C, Deng Q, Zhu L, Liu TC, Duan R, Yang L. Methylene blue pretreatment protects against repeated neonatal isoflurane exposure-induced brain injury and memory loss. Mol Neurobiol. 2024;61(8):5787–801. https://doi.org/10.1007/s12035-024-03931-0. Epub 2024 Jan 17.
3. Apai C, Shah R, Tran K, Pandya Shah S. Anesthesia and the developing brain: a review of sevoflurane-induced neurotoxicity in pediatric populations. Clin Ther. 2021;43(4):762–778. https://doi.org/10.1016/j.clinthera.2021.01.024. Epub 2021 Mar 3. PMID: 33674065.
4. Neag MA, Mitre AO, Catinean A, Mitre CI. An overview on the mechanisms of neuroprotection and neurotoxicity of isoflurane and sevoflurane in experimental studies. Brain Res Bull. 2020;165:281–9. https://doi.org/10.1016/j.brainresbull.2020.10.011. Epub 2020 Oct 17 PMID: 33080307 Review.

Samantha asked around for the opinions of Sophia, and it was almost unanimous that Sophia was a lunatic from a mood disorder as in being Bipolar. They would become partners working hours together. Sophia was tenacious and loved by many. There was never a doubt, however, that Sophia was a "wack job."

"Sam, I have to say I do not believe that exposure to sevoflurane to neonates causes central nervous system damage."

"Sofia!!! How can you say that?" We just started! There are countless investigations since the Consortium paper. Clearly, there are flaws in every investigation. Our role is not to take sides. Our job is to determine what counts as data and what statistical model we choose to analyze the data. The more papers that we review the more data we have. If we do the right thing, we may know the answer to the clinical question. This is not "how you feel" after one flawed paper.! It is a fucking meta analysis! Do you even know what that means? Based on your inability to critically read and impulsiveness, I will talk to Brianna to eliminate you from this study. You are clueless."

"If you talk to Brianna to eliminate me from the study, I will ruin your pathetic life".

Sam had a problem. Sophia would ruin her life. Every threat that Sofia made turned out to be true.

"Sofia, there is a simple solution. Let's have a drink together and I will teach you what we need to do here."

"Thank you Sam! I know a bar that is open right near here"

"I am sure you do and take your meds please."

Suggested Reading

1. Disma N, Withington D, McCann ME, Hunt RW, Arnup SJ, Izzo F, de Graaff JC, Mattioli G, Morton N, Frawley G, Davidson A, Lynn A, Szmuk P, Thomas JJ, Ragg P, Pini Prato A, GAS Consortium. Surgical practice and outcome in 711 neonates and infants undergoing hernia repair in a large multicenter RCT: secondary results from the GAS Study. J Pediatr Surg. 2018;53(9):1643–50. https://doi.org/10.1016/j.jpedsurg.2018.01.003. Epub 2018 Jan 31. PMID: 2960255.
2. McCann ME, de Graaff JC, Dorris L, Disma N, Withington D, Bell G, Grobler A, Stargatt R, Hunt RW, Sheppard SJ, Marmor J, Giribaldi G, Bellinger DC, Hartmann PL, Hardy P, Frawley G, Izzo F, von Ungern Sternberg BS, Lynn A, Wilton N, Mueller M, Polaner DM, Absalom AR, Szmuk P, Morton N, Berde C, Soriano S, Davidson AJ, GAS Consortium. Neurodevelopmental outcome at 5 years of age after general anaesthesia or awake-regional anaesthesia in infancy (GAS): an international, multicentre, randomised, controlled equivalence trial. Lancet. 2019;393(10172):664–77. https://doi.org/10.1016/S0140-6736(18)32485-1. Epub 2019 Feb 14. PMID: 30782342.

Anesthesiologists with Mood Disorders

9

Samantha Dixon, Sofia Gangliano

Sophia was born at a rock concert. She was too young to have been born at Woodstock, but the New Orleans Jazz Festival stood alone in the modern era with 4 days of incredible music, crafts, and, above all, fantastic food.

Her hippie parents did not leave the concert scene even if Sophia's mother came to the Festival with contractions. They packed a bag with all of the necessities in case Sophia was born: warm blankets, sterile scissors, huggies, formula, breast pumps, perfectly white towels, wipes, and sterile water. After Paul Simon and before Santana, Sophia was born after 20 minutes of contractions. There was absolutely no reason not to leave the concert and go to Trinity. Essentially, her father caught her, and no doctor was needed. Her mother's placenta firmed up, and the colostrum showed up by early evening. Sophia started out her life as being "wild" and had a legacy of uncontrollable wildness. She lived the first 2 years of her life on a commune in Oregon and was educated in the public schools in Portland, Oregon.

Sophia was turned off on drugs but not booze. It was in her parent's drug culture, just as her memory was forming, and she wanted no part of it. No weed, cocaine, or H. Beer and wine "did not work for her." She started to hoard hard liquor at the age of 12. Sofia got her first DWI when she was 14. Too young to drink. Too young to drive.

Her first time being expelled but not the last, started in the tenth grade. Sophia lost her mind and beat a teacher to a pulp and was expelled for life. There were no charges filed. Her parents paid for an elite boarding school for young women in Amherst, Massachusetts. The school was structured, and every day was planned with discipline, dignity, and service. During her life of chaos, things went horrifically bad on a flight back to New Orleans. The overhead bin was leaking Tequila onto the passenger on the next seat. The bottle was in the outside pocket of her duffle bag. The devil in her back grew worse when her carton of Marlboros was soaked.

Sofia was brilliant. Without any interest in conventional learning, she was in the 95th percentile on her SATs. She started a hotline for abused women in the Baton

C. Scher, *Anesthesia Conversations*,
https://doi.org/10.1007/978-3-032-05354-1_9

Rouge area, as well as group therapy for women who were victims. She made it known that politically she was from the left. Her social life never included a man or a woman. Sofia was "two dates and done."

Her college application did include a recent DWI and the assault on a teacher.

Would any school want someone so out of control? Sofia was accepted at Louisiana State University in Baton Rouge and at the Trinity School of Medicine in New Orleans. It was not yet settled in her mind whether she wanted to be a physician. She needed to include in her transcript a commitment to her premed requirements. Sofia was able to control her wild streak except for smoking a pack a day and drinking countless bottles of Stoli.

The elite medical schools did not even grant her an interview, and Trinity was her only interview. The thought of going to med school in New Orleans had the potential of doubling her level of questionable poor behavior.

Sofia's activism, energy, and even her criminal acts were a "turn on" for Trinity. While doing well enough for the premed requirements, she had a 4.0 average in her major; philosophy. The new version of Sofia took her studies seriously.

Sofia applied to 30 anesthesiology residencies and was accepted only to Trinity. Sofia needed to dry up, stop smoking, and enter therapy. After 2 months of therapy, she was prescribed Seroquel, Klonopin, and Lamictal. She was relieved that she was diagnosed as being Bipolar. There was a treatment for her mental health issues.

Samantha

A malpractice case that Samantha was loosely involved with had gained traction and now included her. She was complicit in transfusing a Jehovah's Witness patient. Samantha went from under the grid in the department to front and center.

The grind of getting up at 4 AM each morning and getting home at 11 PM, turned her into an insomniac. Samantha could only keep her guard up for so long from the strangling pressure of the cases. Samantha had chosen academic medicine with book deadlines, numerous rejected manuscripts, and teaching her residents giving anesthesia while they were watching social media. Her numerous teaching awards reflected her zeal for education, but it had been 10 years since she received an award or at least some recognition for her work. Among her friends, she was known to cancel dinner reservations when she would stare at her watch and count down the hours that would interrupt her sleep. A psychiatrist diagnosed depression.

Samantha went through Zoloft, Lexapro, and now was on Wellbutrin. She was spending 500 dollars a session in therapy, and she was now on her seventh therapist. A martini did better for her state of mind than therapy.

It is not clear why she came home late every night. She was working on five different projects nightly from lectures, papers, and book chapters to editing a book on pediatric anesthesia. She came home around eleven each night, only to the exasperation of her husband. He raised their son alone, and Sam never showed emotion with her son.

Her husband hired a private detective to determine why Samantha was actually coming home so late. The detective discovered that Samantha was actually working.

Simply stated, Samantha chose her work over her husband and son. After a year of the lifestyle that Sam chose, her husband filed for divorce. The divorce was simple. Because Samantha abandoned her husband and son, she lost everything; her son, house, and all of the expenses related to her son went to her husband. Samantha got nothing. The loss was devastating to her, but she knew that she had earned it. She could not help herself. After days or weeks of the filing, Samantha was relieved. The judge, after all, made it perfectly clear that she was awful as a mother and a wife. At no time had she attempted to improve despite the anguish of her husband. Samantha knew that all of it was true.

Samantha had become wealthy. She knew that one of the formulas to create wealth was not to spend money on shopping, high rents, or buying above her means. There were a few purchases of weed and coke, but they troubled her troubled brain.

She was lucky to have a wealth manager who created a portfolio that allowed her to be free from anesthesia. She questioned herself continuously about whether she had chosen the wrong field of medicine. She no longer liked the practice of anesthesia; disagreements with the surgeons, the lack of respect from residents in different residencies, the lack of true ownership of patients, and hours on end waiting for surgeons operating when there was absolutely nothing to do once the anesthetic was well underway. She was now a burnt pediatric anesthesiologist.

Although she had countless fights with Sofia, they loved each other. They fought their mental health problems together and were always considered invaluable to the department. They vied for the attention from Chris. Sofia intentionally acted like a "wack job." That always attracted attention. Sometimes good but most of the time, bad.

Suggested Reading

1. Bajwa SJ, Jindal R, Kaur J, Singh A. Psychiatric diseases: need for an increased awareness among the anesthesiologists. J Anaesthesiol Clin Pharmacol. 2011;27(4):440–6. https://doi.org/10.4103/0970-9185.86572. PMID: 22096274.
2. Lacy BE, Chan JL. Physician burnout: the hidden health care crisis. Clin Gastroenterol Hepatol. 2018;16(3):311–7. https://doi.org/10.1016/j.cgh.2017.06.043. Epub 2017 Jun 30.PMID: 28669661 Review.
3. Retamal CP, Vandeputte MF, Massman BT. Understanding bipolar disorder: risk factors & protective measures. Rev Med Chil. 2023;151(6):764–74. https://doi.org/10.4067/s0034-98872023000600764. PMID: 38801385 Free article. Review. Spanish.

The Evaluation of Neonatal Hypoxia

10

Samantha Dixon

Samantha's beeper went off at 9 PM. There was a text from Tim Norris. The text said she was needed in the delivery room. Stat!

The newborn was blue despite Tim's ventilating with a mask. The baby's oxygen saturation was so low, the pulse oximeter could not measure the saturation. Tim attempted to intubate twice and did not see vocal cords. Ruby Harris arrived and was able to ventilate with a mask, but like Tim, was not able to visualize the vocal cords. Samantha finally arrived and intubated the baby with one attempt. The EZ-Cap revealed CO2, and the baby's heart rate was now 130 beats. Samantha said nothing. The intubation was rather routine for Sam.

Auscultation was clear, and the bilateral breath sounds were equal on both sides. The endotracheal tube was in the correct position with the tube above the carina. Sam brought up the difficulties of neonatal intubation. The tongue is relatively large, the vocal cords and are anterior when lying flat, and the cords become more anterior due to their relatively large occiput.Ten minutes after the intubation, the baby was blue again. Breath sounds remained bilateral, and the presence of end tidal CO2 was confirmed.

The mother and soon-to-be-born baby were healthy by ultrasound 2 weeks ago. Everything seemed to signal a healthy baby at 37 weeks of gestation. Most non-reassuring fetal heart tracings during labor usually end with a normal baby. The technology of most fetal heart tracings/uterine contractions has not changed in decades.

During her labor, late decelerations strongly suggested neonatal asphyxia, and there was a rush to get the baby out by C-section. The C-section was without complication. The baby boy weighed 7 pounds 3 oz. with an Apgar score or 9/10.

Within 30 minutes, the baby developed tachypnea at 45 breaths per minute. The oxygen saturation was 95. When stimulated, the baby would cry, and his color was a perfect pink. The tachypnea elevated to 50 breaths per minute. Arrangements were made to admit the baby to the neonatal intensive care unit for observation. Samantha was consulted and declared that there are multiple conditions in neonates who start their lives with tachypnea.

C. Scher, *Anesthesia Conversations*,
https://doi.org/10.1007/978-3-032-05354-1_10

Knowledge of neonatal circulation was Samanth's forte. During gestation, the placenta is the location for blood oxygenation which travels to the heart. The pulmonary resistance is so elevated that the oxygenated blood is shunted through the ductus arteriosus (vascular connection from the pulmonary artery and the aorta) and probe patent foramen ovale. At birth, with lung expansion, the pulmonary vascular resistance falls, the ductus closes from oxygenation, and the patent foramen ovale closes in response to blood filling the right ventricle. The newborn went from a parallel circulation to a series circulation. Acidosis, low blood pressure, and cool ambient temperature are among the factors that can cause the series circulation to return to a parallel or fetal circulation that leads to hypoxia.

It was clear that the diagnosis was initially consistent with neonatal transient tachypnea of the newborn. There was no cyanosis, no regression to the fetal circulation, and was apparently a healthy baby. Since the delivery was without the "squeeze" of the birth canal, the water that filled the alveoli missed the physiological squeeze to unburden the amniotic fluid that remained in the lungs. It is not accompanied by hypoxia. This resolves on the first day of life and rarely results in endotracheal intubation.

The baby was transferred to the NICU by Samantha and Tim. Upon arrival at the Neonatal ICU, the baby was blue. The neonatologist, Sam, and Tim had seen this countless times. The new series circulation reversed itself back to a transitional circulation that evolved to a neonatal parallel circulation. The ductus reopened, and the foramen ovale closed.

The list of causes of newborn cyanosis is almost exhaustive; a lack of surfactant in the premature baby, meconium aspiration, pulmonary hypoplasia, diaphragmatic hernia, and congenital heart disease (CHD).

The nomenclature of congenital heart diseases includes all those starting with letter T. The classic mnemonic, the "five T's" of cyanotic congenital heart disease, continues to be useful.

Transposition of the great arteries (TGA), tetralogy of Fallot, truncus arteriosus, total anomalous pulmonary venous connection (TAPVC), and tricuspid valve abnormalities (TVA). The babies that survive these conditions have some mixing of arterialized blood and venous blood. These diseases do not typically declare themselves in the early newborn period. The exception here was a hypoplastic heart. (the most dreaded congenital heart disease that does not begin with T).

Meconium is passed from the colon during hypoxic moments of labor. There is a wide variation of aspirations from brown watery aspiration to thick meconium aspiration. The dreaded thick meconium aspiration interferes with gas exchange as meconium fills multiple bronchi down to alveolar sacs. The result is an overwhelming increase in the pulmonary vascular resistance. The series neonatal circulation can transition to a parallel neonatal circulation which could persist depending on the thickness and volume of meconium aspirated. There is actually some debate surrounding the treatment of meconium aspiration.

Infant Respiratory Distress Syndrome is a lack of surfactant, causing alveolar collapse. There has been significant progress as synthetic surfactants enter the baby through the endotracheal tube. Although no differences were noted between

Survanta- and Exosurf-treated infants regarding the primary outcome of death or chronic lung disease at 28 days of age, the significant improvement in secondary clinical outcomes suggests that Survanta is more effective than Exosurf Neonatal in the treatment of established RDS. Anesthesiologists need the neonatal literature to deliver the best therapeutics in the operating room. Samantha was requested to take care of these babies in the operating room.

Pulmonary hypoplasia is rarely encountered by the anesthesiologist; the distance from the alveoli and pulmonary circulation is significantly too much for gas exchange and is usually a fatal diagnosis in the extremely premature neonate (less than 27 weeks).

Sam was the last person to pat herself on the back. During her pediatric anesthesia fellowship and pediatric critical care fellowship, she became "fluent" with pediatric cardiac ultrasound. The baby was flipping between the desired series circulation into the parallel circulation. The heart and lungs were both normal. There was no other reason for the flip in circulation other than hypothermia. Samantha warmed up the neonate, and the episodes of cyanosis never returned. The baby went to the regular nursery and was discharged the following day with the mother.

Sam did what she was trained to do and did not understand that most anesthesiologists without a pediatric fellowship could not "save the day." That is just the way she is wired. Every field of medicine becomes routine. For Samantha, this was just part of her routine that included high levels of expectation and anxiety. Sam felt a case of burnout was facing her. She hoped that the research project that Brianna proposed would reinvigorate her.

Suggested Reading

1. Finnemore A, Groves A. Physiology of the fetal and transitional circulation. Semin Fetal Neonatal Med. 2015;20(4):210–6. https://doi.org/10.1016/j.siny.2015.04.003. Epub 2015.
2. Friedman AH, Fahey JT. The transition from fetal to neonatal circulation: normal responses and implications for infants with heart disease. Semin Perinatol. 1993;17(2):106–21.
3. Scott M, Neal AE. Congenital heart disease. Prim Care. 2021;48(3):351–66. https://doi.org/10.1016/j.pop.2021.04.005. Epub 2021 Jul 8. PMID: 34311844 Review.
4. Sehgal A, Allison BJ, Miller SL, Polglase GR, McNamara PJ, Hooper SB. Impact of acute and chronic hypoxia-ischemia on the transitional circulation. Pediatrics. 2021;147(3):e2020.
5. Seri I, Noori S. Fetal and neonatal hemodynamics. Semin Fetal Neonatal Med. 2015;20(4):209. https://doi.org/10.1016/j.siny.2015.04.002. Epub 2015 Apr 25. PMID: 25921754.

Malignant Hyperthermia 11

Ruby Harris

Ruby was an only child, and her early childhood dream was to be a pediatrician. She landed on the pathway of her parents' wishes and embraced activism in all of its forms. It started with Meals on Wheels and raised money door by door. She raised money for those physicians and nurses who volunteered to repair cleft lips and palates for children in Africa. She embraced movements that protected voter's rights, the eradication of gun violence, and opposed gerrymandering districts to suppress black voters.

Ruby embraced Black Like Matters, and above all, investigations to determine why black women and other women of color have significantly higher peripartum death rates than white women.

Ruby's undergraduate transcript was excellent except for a D in calculus and a D in organic chemistry. She thought that her calling for pediatrics was over. Her "D"s were not from not trying. Simply, Ruby studied and just did not "get it" in those courses that were a must for premed applicants. She was not on track for a medical school in the United States. Ruby applied to US medical schools, osteopathic schools, and medical schools in Mexico.

She went to her advisor at Tulane, who suggested she meet with Chris Landry at Trinity, who could dump the Ds and replace them with her incredible activism. Chris made sure that she was going to be accepted to the Trinity School of Medicine.

In Ruby's fourth year of medical school, Chris invited Ruby to spend a day in the Department of Anesthesia and a dinner at Brigstens. Ruby never even considered anesthesia. She "avoided" the elective at Trinity. Chris convinced Ruby that a pediatric anesthesiologist was better in every way than pediatricians with critical care boards. Ruby was accepted to the Trinity anesthesia residency in an outside-the-match position.

After 4 years of anesthesia training that included several months of pediatric anesthesia rotations, Ruby was accepted to the pediatric anesthesia fellowship at Emory in Atlanta. She never knew that Chris secured her spot. After 5 years of service as an attending at Emory, Ruby earned 5 teaching awards, authored several

C. Scher, *Anesthesia Conversations*,
https://doi.org/10.1007/978-3-032-05354-1_11

chapters in pediatric anesthesia textbooks, and became the Assistant Program Director at Emory. Chris recruited her to return to Trinity with a promotion to an Associate Professor level. She became the Assistant Director of Pediatric Anesthesia.

Chris's goal was to have half the faculty white and the other with people of color. Over time, his goal was met. Ruby's knowledge of pediatrics and pediatric anesthesia was the best in NOLA.

A four-year-old boy presented for a tonsillectomy and adenoidectomy. His past medical history was significant for chronic infections in his tonsils. The child had never had anesthesia in his past. He was not on any medications and had no drug allergies. His mother had an epidural for a knee surgery, and there was no history of problems related to anesthesia.

The plan for the induction of anesthesia was similar to most of the pediatric inductions; breathe the child down with a mask of sevoflurane. Within seconds, the signs of malignant hyperthermia were apparent to Ruby. After 5 minutes, the child's temperature was 38.5 and his heart rate was 150 beats per minute. Severe jaw rigidity set in. A nurse called for the MH cart, and Ruby secured a 20-gauge IV into the left antecubital fossa. Thirty milligrams of rocuronium and a TIVA with dexmedetomidine, propofol, and remifentanil replaced sevoflurane. A Mapleson D circuit replaced the anesthesia machine that was pushed out of the room. The circuit was attached to the wall oxygen.

Lily and her resident arrived. Lily assigned the resident to intubate, and Lily secured a right radial arterial line. Ruby was working on the Ryanodex. A stat page for the entire department was activated by Lily. Marco walked the ABG over to the cardiac surgery operating room, where there was an ABG analyzer.

The surgeons thought it was premature to label the case as MH and administer dantrolene. Ruby transformed herself into a belligerent monster when a rebuttal to a surgeon's comments that had to be made. By the two-minute mark, Ryanodex (dantrolene) was ready for administration. The signs of MH were now fully apparent; an increase in ETCO2, rectal temperature of 40 degrees Celsius, tachycardia, masseter muscle spasm, and a mixed respiratory and metabolic acidosis on ABG.

Ruby with rushed speech asked, what is next? Ruby remained on course with her sound decision to act with the administration of dantrolene ASAP.

The focus of attention was no longer on the patient. It was on Ruby. An anesthesia lesson was dumbed down and directed at the pediatric surgeons. Ruby was multitasking in the care of the child. Ruby took no shit from anyone. She was giving her iconic lecture on malignant hyperthermia.

"Ryanodine receptors form a class of calcium channels or simply 'tunnels'. The RYR2 ryanodine receptor is the major cellular mediator of receptor induced calcium release. The receptor is on the 'walls' of the sarcoplasmic reticulum and in MH susceptible people, these receptors are abnormal. With triggering agents (inhalational anesthetics, succinylcholine), ryanodine receptors cannot control the intracellular sarcoplasmic reticulum release calcium into the cytosol, leading to damage of the cell wall and cell death. The surgery was canceled and a call for help for other anesthesiologists was made. The malignant hyperthermia cart and the online directions by MHAUS were now on the computer screen that served initially as the EMR.

A cooling blue rubber water-filled blanket was placed under the child. Ryanodex (2.5 mg/kg) was administered, and there was a significant improvement, but clearly the child was "not out of the woods." A second dose of dantrolene at 5 mg/kg was repeated 5 minutes after the first dose. A repeat ABG revealed a normalizing acid/base status and decreasing potassium levels. The body temperature was down from 39 degrees to 38.0. Blood samples were sent for CPK and urine for myoglobinuria. The child was extubated when all labs normalized, and the usual signs of extubation criteria were met. The child was transported to the pediatric intensive care unit and was somewhat agitated and mildly weak from the two doses of dantrolene. There was a notable difference in opinion among the pediatric intensive care unit's attendings about continuing dantrolene dosing.

Ruby had developed an unbreakable poor opinion of the pediatricians. "We need to follow the recommendations of MAUS." Plain and simple This is not the time for innovation. I bet you all have not seen MH and yet, you had doubts about this being the real thing. To be clear, this is malignant hyperthermia. Period.

"MHAUS (Malignant Hyperthermia Association of the United States) recommends continuing maintenance doses of dantrolene 1 mg/kg intravenous IV bolus every 4 to 6 hours or 0.25 mg/kg/hour IV continuous infusion) for at least 24 hours after the last observed sign of MH. Recrudescence of MH occurs in approximately 20% of patients after initial treatment, at a mean of 13 hours after the initial reaction. If recurrent signs appear in spite of ongoing treatment additional dantrolene boluses may be required."

Ruby suggested, when the child was stable and ready for discharge, to the parents that the family go for susceptibility testing; genetic testing. A gene change (mutation) that makes one susceptible to malignant hyperthermia is identified using genetic testing. A sample of blood is collected and sent to a lab for analysis.Genetic testing can now be used to isolate those at risk for malignant hypothermia.

A muscle biopsy test is the gold (contracture test) standard for malignant hyperthermia. In most cases, healthcare providers recommend a muscle biopsy if one is at risk of malignant hyperthermia. During this test, a small piece of muscle tissue is surgically removed for lab analysis. In the lab, the specimen is exposed to triggering chemicals hyperthermia to determine how the muscle contracts. Because this test must be done on muscle tissue immediately after removing it, travel to a specialized muscle biopsy center is necessary.

Testing challenges parents, as fresh tissue usually means airline tickets, hotels, meals, and taxis. Marco and Anne gave their suggestion to simply label the child as an MH patient. This would avoid the expenses of tests that do have false positives and negatives and make it simple, if he came for any surgery in the future. Ruby was upset with Marco's and Anne's suggestion but now understood the practicality of just calling the child MH prone for his life.

Ruby wanted to present another case. Being a detective for her next case required some understanding of the first case: A five-year-old female presented to the emergency room 48 hours after bilateral strabismus repair. Her medical history was significant for juvenile diabetes mellitus which was controlled with insulin. In the emergency room, she was tachypneic, diaphoretic, and agitated. Her blood pressure was 160/90, heart rate 130, and temperature of 104 degrees. Her mother said these symptoms started an hour ago. The first 24 hours after surgery were without incident. The mother was present for the inhalational induction with sevoflurane. She was escorted out of the operating room and into the PACU when the case was over. There was minimal pain, no PONV, and blood sugars were between 90 and 110 during her short stay in the ambulatory surgical center. The child had a full dinner and was asleep by 8 o'clock PM the day of surgery.

The pediatric emergency physician ordered a basic metabolic panel: ABG, lactate, CPK, and urine for myoglobin. The thought process in this case was simple. MH cannot start more than 4 hours after triggering anesthetics DKA was ruled out with a normal ABG.

Marco, Anne, and Olive were sure that MH was the problem. Ruby disagreed, but the pediatric attending did not see any reason to hold back on dantrolene administration and follow the MHAUS guidelines. Ruby could not disagree more.

"MH does not present this way; hours after the surgery with the patient well at home!. Chris came down and always supported his faculty, in this case Ruby. The CPK and ABG would resolve the dispute."

"MH is the diagnosis. What else could this be?" Marco, with minimal experience, was firm that nothing else could explain this?

Ruby had seen 10 cases in her career and was current with her reading. "Ok, late MH can occur but it is super rare; less than 0.1%. If it was more than rare, we would be keeping patients in the hospitals for days. The danger of late onset MH is that there would be significant time lapse from diagnosis and treatment."

"This is not MH.! The labs came back in an hour and were totally normal. Ruby said no more. There was no explanation for this. Wait! Let me rephrase what I just said. There is a reason for this, It is just that we have not found it. I do not think that giving a dose of Ryanodex poses any significant risk. It is excellent for fever, We will admit him to the pediatric intensive care unit, simply for observation."

The pediatric patient stayed one night. All repeat labs were normal including the CPK. He was discharged, and Ruby gave detailed instructions to the family if symptoms recurred. Ruby called the mother at five in the afternoon and just before midnight. The child was fine and playing with his toys.

Suggested Reading

1. Ellinas H, Albrecht MA. Malignant hyperthermia update. Anesthesiol Clin. 2020;38(1):165–81. https://doi.org/10.1016/j.anclin.2019.10.010. PMID: 32008650 Review.
2. Hopkins PM, Girard T, Dalay S, Jenkins B, Thacker A, Patteril M, McGrady E. Malignant hyperthermia 2020: guideline from the Association of Anaesthetists. Anaesthesia. 2021;76(5):655–64. https://doi.org/10.1111/anae.15317. Epub 2021 Jan 5.
3. Lawal TA, Todd JJ, Meilleur KG. Ryanodine receptor 1-related myopathies: diagnostic and therapeutic approaches. Neurotherapeutics. 2018;15(4):885–99. https://doi.org/10.1007/s13311-018-00677-1.
4. Rosenberg H, Pollock N, Schiemann A, Bulger T, Stowell K. Malignant hyperthermia: a review. J Rare Dis. 2015;10:93. https://doi.org/10.1186/s13023-015-0310-1. PMID: 26238698 Free PMC article. Review.

The Perils of Office-Based Anesthesia 12

Gilbert Lau

Gill was in a rut. He had, at baseline, paranoia. He believed that his daily assignments of his cases at Trinity assigned to have him fail. He resigned from Trinity and took a position in a plastic surgeon's office to provide anesthesia for cosmetic surgery. The challenging office-based cosmetic surgeries were on his days; Monday, Tuesday, and Thursday. He was one of two anesthesiologists in a 3 "OR" office. Five plastic surgeons owned the office. They were all over the age of 65 and operated exclusively at the office. They could only use Gil in one OR at a time. Cosmetic cases normally lasted for hours with this geriatric group of surgeons.

The group collected the anesthesia bills and gave Gil a salary from those collections. The group gave 450,000 dollars a year with full benefits. His hours were 7–3 plus overtime at 350 dollars per hour. The salary, benefits, and hours were exactly what he was looking for. Gil never complained but expressed concerns regarding safety. He knew that the business was making a "killing" from the anesthesia bills, but felt fortunate for his business arrangement.

Plastic surgery was a cash business, and Gil planned at the 6-month mark of his employment time to ask for a raise. He could not imagine why this lucrative group of surgeons would turn his request down. He believed that the surgeons could not find someone better to replace him.

It was a "primo" job for the nursing staff and scrub techs. Their salaries were higher than a job of the same title in New Orleans. They were loyal to the surgeons and did not care what Gil was concerned about.. They did not want to rock the boat. They wanted their paycheck and knew that they were simply paid more for their jobs at any other site in the city.

Gil made no attempt to control his building hatred of his predicament. The end was always the same for him. He had several jobs over the years, but always let his mood degenerate over time at every job he worked on. He was mad at the world.

Overtime, the staff viewed him as being toxic. The last three anesthesiologists lasted less than 3 weeks, but these reasons for leaving were never about the job: divorce, drug addiction by a son, and a wife displaced from her job.

C. Scher, *Anesthesia Conversations*,
https://doi.org/10.1007/978-3-032-05354-1_12

Gill was acutely aware that he was losing his significant anesthesia skills over time. The cases he was assigned to never needed a central line, a nerve blocks an arterial line or Swan-Ganz catheter. If they were in need of such procedures, the case would be have to be done in a hospital. He missed the camaraderie of the anesthesia and surgery physicians. Gil posted his profile on Indeed. He gave himself a quitting or else date: 1 month away.

There was an outpatient surgery center owned by a business-savvy Korean woman, one block away from Baptist Hospital. Diane Lee also owned a surgical center on Prytania, just past Washington, with eight operating rooms, and another in the Quarter on Burgundy, just off Bourbon Street, with five operating rooms. Gil wondered why there was a surgical center in the French Quarter. Parking was a nightmare, and the office had a weird layout. Gil believed the space was not suitable for a residence or a business. He took another leap of faith, and Diane signed him up on Gil's last day of anesthesia at the office-based surgery

The sole owner of this business was Diane, who set up a limo system where a limo would go to the residence of the patients and transport them to the surgery center. The patients were driven to their homes upon discharge. This service, while impressive, was built into a very padded bill. She had fresh flowers and sushi for families who were in the waiting room. Diane converted the "house" into 5 operating rooms. In addition, there was a space for a PACU, consultation room, and an infusion center for all infusion medications except cancer treatments. There was still room for an extravagant two-bedroom apartment which became the waiting room. Diane Lee was neither a physician nor in the medical field. She was a business major at Emory and earned her Master's in Business at LSU.

Gil's employment would not improve his fading anesthesia skills, but the pay was more than he had in his career. He had not done this kind of work before and assumed that safety related to anesthesia was strictly adhered to.

Ryanodex, intralipid, a crash cart with a working defibrillator, emergency drugs, and video laryngoscopes were a must. There had to be a seamless plan to move patients out of the surgery center to the hospital if need be. Gil was satisfied with what he was told and listened intently. He never actually looked in the "workroom area" to verify what was told to him.

In surgery centers with anesthesia and surgery, rigorous credentialing, verification of board certification, malpractice history, and proof of continuing education are often lacking. Record keeping and reporting complications were a must, but more often than not, they were not reported. There was no documentation of any adverse effects due to anesthesia. This was not the case in Diane Lee's centers.

Diane, with a business first mentality, was impeccable with proper credentialing, vetting of physicians and nurses, scrub techs, and outsourced maintenance workers. She followed every regulation. The plan was to utilize Gil's experience and expertise to make anesthesia a model for safety and efficiency among the many New Orleans surgicenters. Diane made an investment of purchasing an EMR that improved patient center care and increase billing.

The majority of the cases were sports related. A comprehensive pre-op evaluation was always in the electronic medical record. Julie was meticulous about documentation. An anesthesiologist will leave the office when a patient is ready to leave. Diane was all about "doing the right thing". As the sole owner, Diane did not have to justify her business decisions. Cutting profits by investing in technology made sense to her. Hiring Gill as a 1099 gave her a false sense of protection.

Gil was at peace working in the Vieux Carre (French Quarter). Knee arthroscopies with repair or removal of a meniscus, bunionectomies, and most hernias, comprised most of the cases. Neuraxial anesthesia, patients whose BMI was above 32, pregnant patients, and children below the age of 15, could not be operated on at the surgery center.

A McGrath video scope was dedicated for all intubations. A hand-held ultrasound for difficult venous access and peripheral nerve blocks added efficiency and efficacy of anesthesiology. Gil's crash course in nerve blocks made him current. The surgeons never said no to a request for a device that increased their success and safety. Gil let the surgeons know that the only LMA stocked was the I-Gel. After 1 month, Gil had succeeded in stabilizing his mood.

A 27-year-old skier with no medical problems presented for, a repair of a completely torn meniscus. The anesthesia induction was with propofol and rocuronium and maintained with sevoflurane and oxygen. The surgeon did not want a nerve block prior to the induction of anesthesia. The endotracheal intubation was easy. Diane did not want to deal with the DEA. There were no controlled substances, and there was enough local anesthesia in the case to ensure a close to zero pain score while recovering in the PACU.

At the eight-minute mark past induction and just after the intubation, Gil's first patient of the day became tachycardic and extremely hypertensive; 189/110. The esophageal stethoscope temperature measured 39 degrees Celsius. Gil went straight to the conclusion that this was malignant hyperthermia. He wished there were a blood gas machine, but there was not. He needed a vial of Ryanodex to start, but there was no Ryanodex at the surgery center. He told the office manager to call for an ambulance STAT. Gil screamed into the phone and ordered the ED nurses at the affiliated hospital to load up the ambulance with at least 10 vials of dantrolene or Ryanodex. Every minute of delay would lead to a death. Gil could not predict when the EMT would arrive.

EMT arrived 3 minutes after the original phone call and brought only one vial of Ryanodex. With a dose of 2.5/kg, one ampule of 250 mg would be enough for the moment.

"What the fuck! I said I needed 10 vials, not one! Each vial of Ryanodex had 250 mg of Dantrolene, with sterile water. The dose for the moment was 2.5 mg/kg. or 200 mg of a vial of 250 mg."

"Holy shit! How is it possible for one vial? What the fuck! Where is the ambulance? The clock was ticking. Gil found some lasix and gave the whole vial of 40 mg. Gil set up a propofol infusion on a pump when EMS arrived. They were supposed to have brought more Ryanodex but their was a total lack of communication. Diane appointed Gil to raise the bar for anesthesia and he failed. While he was told that there was Ryanodex, he never went into the work room to check on the supply.

"We have to leave ASAP. We have no time to wait for the Ryanodex! We are going now"! Gil thought that hyperkalemia and control of acid/ base balance were urgent and started to treat these threats that could end her life. Hyperventilation drove potassium into the cells. An amp of calcium would protect the heart. Cooling her down was essential. Sheets with cold water, instead of ice, covered the patient."

The patient was transported with a pump syringe of propofol and ventilated with the only Ambu bag that was in the center. The ride of 5 minutes felt like an hour, and Gil had radioed the hospital emergency room to get at least 10 vials of Ryanodex ready for their arrival. As they passed through the emergency entry door, the EKG on the transport monitor was flat line. CPR began.

One milligram of epinephrine was administered and CPR continued. A femoral pulse was not palpable, and the monitor was now showing ventricular fibrillation. This was a shockable rhythm, and a shock was given. The new rhythm was sinus tachycardia. Her blood pressure was 72/34. One ampule of calcium chloride and 250 mg of Ryanodex were administered. An arterial line was started, and a blood gas was drawn and handed off to a nurse who had the code to run the ABG. The pH was 7.12, potassium 6.7, and lactate 8. Norepinephrine was put on a pump at 8 mcg, and the vasopressin infusion pump was activated. A bag of normal saline was pouring into the patient and a glucose/insulin infusion was initiated.

Within minutes, the blood pressure rose to 130/85. Her sinus tachycardia became a normal sinus rhythm, and palpable pulses were felt in both grounds. The norepinephrine was stopped, and the next arterial pH was 7.31 with a potassium level of 6.2. Her lactate had come down to 3. The Ryanodex was clearly working. The patient was transported to the medical ICU. They chose to give an infusion of Ryanodex for 24 hours. She was ready for extubation by 10 PM. The CPK was 8000 mcg/liter.

The patient came close to death. Diane Lee and her attorneys proceeded with a RCA on the case. At times, the discussion became very heated. A decision was made. One of the most essential chores that an anesthesiologist has is to check and count every day the cabinet where drugs are kept. There was no cart dedicated to MH. The ability of the surgery center to perform ACLS was limited. Essential medications were not in the surgery center. Gil brought his own video-scope. There was no backup, if Gil's was broken. There was an expired vial of ketamine in the cabinet for 2 years. Why did the owners of the center not take ownership of the inadequate items that are essential for safe anesthesia? There were no narcotics for pain after surgery? Why was the message to bring more Ryanodex a failure of communication?

The deficiencies were targeted at Gil. Undoubtedly, he did not check out the stocking of the dantrolene or several other medications that were "musts" but were not present in the surgery center. Gil assumed when he walked in the door that these successful surgeons had done what it takes to make the procedure safe. Gil wanted to know if the previous anesthesiologist restocked the cart every day. He did. Gil did not believe them. Gil, by nature, was meticulous about his work, and he more than dropped the ball in this case. He did not check if the essentials of anesthesia practice were in the office.

The family of the patient received a summary of the critical events and the plan for change. They hired an attorney for legal action. After a comprehensive investigation, Gill was guilty of negligence. The family's only demand was to fire Gil and report Gil to the Division of Professional Licensing in Louisiana and the OPC (Office of Professional Conduct).

Gill went for a plea. Gil would be terminated from the practice, and there would be a suspension of his medical license for 6 months. This event would be on the State Licensing Website. The judge mulled over his sentence. He thought losing his license could put an end to Gil's life as a physician. The judge did not want to end Gil's career. Against the overbearing wishes of the family, the judge amended his original sentence. Under this new sentence, Gil's license was not suspended, but he could not practice medicine for 6 months in the State of Louisiana. The questions came up too many times, "Why did he not check for the adequate stocking of Ryanodex? What else was missing?"

It takes 4 months to receive credentials after agreeing to take a position. It takes two or more months of interviewing for positions. There was a total of 6 months of not earning a paycheck, and Gil was relieved by how the events unfolded. He could go without a paycheck for years, but there was an urgency to become a doctor again.

Gil applied to over 100 departments. He assumed that his crisis had spread all over social media and at anesthesia meetings both in the United States and internationally. Gil had an attorney to guide him down the path to make him whole again. They composed a personal statement that had clarity and introspection. The statement worked. Gil was able to secure 25 interviews. He was offered three positions. He said "yes" to the first program that offered him a job. The legendary John H. Stroger Hospital of Cook County offered him a full-time faculty position at Rush University.

The attorney reminded Gil that every instinct he had surrounding this case was wrong. Gil was locked into his attorney for the rest of his professional life. His attorney asked for 50,000 a year, and Gil was thrilled to pay it.

Gil's lack of attention to detail almost ended up in the death of a patient. He had girlfriends that ended quickly for 5 years. Hours of therapy restored him. Gil became a full Professor and was the site Director of Anesthesiology at Cook County and married to the first cousin of his attorney. The payments stopped.

Suggested Reading

1. Coldiron B, Shreve E, Balkrishnan R. Patient injuries from surgical procedures performed in medical offices: three years of Florida data. Dermatol Surg. 2004;30(12 Pt 1):1435–43. https://doi.org/10.1111/j.1524-4725.2004.30500.x; discussion 1443. PMID: 15606728.
2. Osman BM, Shapiro FE. Office-Based anesthesia: a comprehensive review and 2019 update. Anesthesiol Clin. 2019;37(2):317–31. https://doi.org/10.1016/j.anclin.2019.01.004. Epub 2019 Mar 22. PMID: 31047132 Review.
3. Seligson E, Beutler SS, Urman RD. Office-based anesthesia: an update on safety and outcomes (2017-2019). Curr Opin Anaesthesiol. 2019;32(6):756–61. https://doi.org/10.1097/ACO.0000000000000789. PMID: 31483329 Review.

Pediatric PTSD

13

Marco Colleta

The career that one chooses must be sustainable. The requirements that make a career sustainable are those that do not cause physical damage to patients or long episodes of mental health illness. The career must excite you as the years go on. The fact that if one had "enough" by age 45, the path chosen implies that the field of medicine chosen was not sustainable. A sustainable choice is one that you can see yourself engaged in a field that will take you to retirement with some level of enthusiasm and mental immersion.

Well into his anesthesia residency, there were significant moments when Marco Colleta saved lives. The first case of the morning would be very exciting, and the second case could go on for hours with not much to do. There were too many days after the induction and intubation that were simply downtime. In December of his final year of anesthesia residency, his mind turned 180 degrees and chose to do a second residency in Psychiatry. Marco Colleta made the decision to finish the process of becoming a board certified in Anesthesiology. Lily and Chris were stunned. Chris wanted him on the faculty.

Marco made an appointment with the Program Director and Chairman of the Department of Psychiatry at Trinity. The department was only two floors above the Department of Anesthesiology. All of the elite departments that received his CV and wanted to arrange a FaceTime interview. Trinity asked him to come up the two flights of stairs ASAP. Within 15 minutes of his meeting, he signed a contract.

The psychiatry residency gave Marco credit for his anesthesiology. He did not need a medical internship and was able to jump right into psychiatry. Psychiatry was always his passion, but he had been "talked out of it" because of the shitty income that was part of the life of a "shrink". Marco knew how not to have a shitty income.

Marco grew up in New York City. His parents divorced when Marco was four, and his father had full custody of him. Marco has no memory of his mother. His mother entered the marriage with a hidden addiction to alcohol and cocaine. Her illness was transparent in the first year of her marriage. Marco's father did everything conceivable to get her sober, but her physical abuse of Marco was the last

C. Scher, *Anesthesia Conversations*,
https://doi.org/10.1007/978-3-032-05354-1_13

straw. To this day, Marco and his father know nothing about her present life. Marco's father is grateful that Marco has no memory of her.

Marco was the quintessential nerd until he entered high school. He was married to his XBOX, and he was socially inept. He went to Hunter College and graduated magna cum laude in his major in mathematics. His academic performance was pristine, and he excelled in his major. He chose Columbia for Medical School among six other schools that accepted him. He wanted a program that was research and science-heavy. In the days when the USMLE score was everything for resident training programs, Marco scored a 252. It is a high score that hardly anyone can achieve. Somewhere during his medical school, he migrated to anesthesia.

A weekend at the New Orleans Jazz and Heritage Festival, and dinners at Galatoire's and Commander's Palace started the warm spot in his wife, Lena and Marco's hearts about New Orleans. A visit to the schools for his boys and the possibility of owning a Victorian home in "Uptown" could not be beat. The Colletas embraced New Orleans one hundred percent.

The Coletta family were foodies, and the price was right for the Andouille Crusted Fish pan, house-made andouille breadcrumbs, carrot and mirliton batons, and Crab Ravigote. Lena did not like Bechamel and Hollandaise sauce. That changed quickly after a few meals with those unique to New Orleans flavors. They admitted they loved the crazy culture of parties, and the ease of making friends were enticing.

Marco accepted the out-of-the-match spot offered by Chris. His wife, Lena, was on the faculty of Tulane and on the professor track in History. Lena was editing her dissertation for her PhD. and like Marco, was considering a career 180; law school. With Marco's new career and his wife's possible law school, their paths were not terribly disruptive to the boys. The big plan was to raise the boys in New Orleans. The steep cost of the Newman School was worth taking a loan. This was the first and only loan that Marco needed. It gave them breathing room.

The boys were happy, and "do not wake the sleeping dog" was their philosophy of parenting. They were all in on staying in NOLA and spent hours finding their own home. They bought a home on Jefferson Ave, only blocks from The Newman School.

Marco was attracted to science, technology, and procedural skills that led to adrenaline rushes when he was successful in cases that challenged him. He became a fan favorite among the faculty members with his work ethic and the bonds that he formed with his patients. He was voted Best Resident of the Year in his final year of anesthesia residency. His psychiatry secret blossomed at the end of his CA-1 year when he was bombarded with the many negatives of the culture of anesthesiology. He went to medical school to become a "healer" and that sentiment was not part of anesthesiology.

When the surgeons made a request, he or she addressed "Hey Anesthesia" as if anesthesiologists were not physicians. Every resident had a twenty-minute coffee break in the morning, a thirty-minute lunch break, and then another coffee break in the mid-afternoon. The surgeons were always engaged with their cases and rarely took breaks, even if they operated for hours. There was an EMR on a computer that included every medication, vital sign, and procedure automatically displayed on the computer screen. When a surgical case became outright boring (septal rhinoplasty), Marco and his fellow residents would click on the chrome icon. It was time to shop on Amazon, make travel arrangements, or simply check the inbox for emails. The breaks, coupled with online trip reservations to Hawaii, made attending surgeons and the surgical residents apoplectic. "These guys are generating enormous bills for their patients by shopping!".

Marco Colleta stood out as a resident who verbally was against all of the breaks and all of the behaviors that were inherent to anesthesia. "Enough"!

Marco had one last case in his anesthesia residency.

A 7-year old girl was scheduled for dental restoration. She needed seven teeth removed and four root canals. Her father accompanied her to the preop office and said that she was in good health.

Up until this case, Marco had done very few pediatric cases. His patient was in the holding area and was screaming and crying at the highest possible decibel level. Her father barely could restrain her. She refused to wear the hospital pajamas and remained in street clothes.

Marco's first inclination was oral midazolam. After 10 minutes, the child was not sedated and ramped up her hysteria. Marco proceeded with a combination of midazolam and ketamine, again orally. It remained a "No go." Nasal dexmedetomidine did not touch her. She was hysterical to the point that her nose was filled with secretions, and any attempt to calm her down increased her hysteria.

Marco then planned for the "atomic bomb" of sedation. Marco injected ketamine: 4 mg/kg, intramuscularly, directly through the pajama legs. The father's job was to keep the child's arms from grabbing Marco's arms during the shot. The technique of the injection was perfect. Nystagmus of the eyes was one of the signs of ketamine that usually preceded sleep. The father carried the sleeping patient and child to the operating room. Marco felt successful and, at the same time, dismayed that something was missing in this case.

As monitors were applied in the operating room, the child woke up! Marco was more than incredulous as this was not how he wanted his last case to play out. The father and Marco decided that the case should be postponed until a better approach was offered. An hour was needed for observation due to the polypharmacy administered. Marco apologized to the father.

The father did say that his daughter had not been the same since she came to the States. The family lived in Aleppo during the Syrian Civil War. Aleppo experienced intense bombardments, including those by the Assad regime, leading to widespread destruction and civilian casualties. During the bombings and the child witnessed the death of some friends and family. This was a case of PTSD which matched the behavior of the child.

Marco had a plan he had read about. The child had to be desensitized. This was a five-day plan. The child, father, and Marco would spend 15 minutes in an empty operating room, allowing the child to walk around the operating room, seeing and touching objects. The next 3 days progressed to allowing a facemask on her face. By day five, she was ready for an inhalational induction and did not need a premedication. Marco beat himself up that he did not recognize PTSD. Marco's legacy was growing.

Suggested Reading

1. De Young AC, Landolt MA. PTSD in children below the age of 6 years. Curr Psychiatry Rep. 2018;20(11):97. https://doi.org/10.1007/s11920-018-0966.
2. Eijlers R, Dierckx B, Staals LM, Berghmans JM, van der Schroeff MP, Strabbing EM, Wijnen RMH, Hillegers MHJ, Legerstee JS. Virtual reality exposure before elective day care surgery to reduce anxiety and pain in children: a randomised controlled trial. Eur J Anaesthesiol. 2019;36(10):728–37. https://doi.org/10.1097/EJA.0000000000001059.
3. Gao J, Wang F, Wang X, Zou X, Liu HC, Song X, Chai X, Jiang R, Zhao P, Zhang J, Wang SY, Ma H, Zhao Z, Wang Q, Zhou N, Bai J, Zhang J. Safety and efficacy of a novel dexmedetomidine nasal spray for preanesthetic sedation in children: a randomized, double-blind, placebo-controlled trial. BMC Anesthesiol. 2024;24(1):315. https://doi.org/10.1186/s12871-024-02708-1. PMID: 39242499.
4. Rahimi MP, Wafa MH, Stanikzai MH, Rahimi BA. Post-traumatic stress disorder (PTSD) probability among parents who live in Kandahar, Afghanistan and lost at least a child to armed conflict. Sci Rep. 2023;13(1):3994. https://doi.org/10.1038/s41598-023-31228-0.
5. Smith P, Perrin S, Tim D, Meiser-Stedman R, Clark DM, Yule W. Treatment of posttraumatic stress disorder in children and adolescents. Curr Opin Psychiatry. 2013;26(1):66–72.

Arrhythmogenic Right Ventricular Cardiomyopathy

14

Olivia Jordan

Olivia Jordan was not Olivia Jordan when she was born. Due to rising racism against Muslims in the United States, her parents legally changed the name of everyone in the immediate family from Ali to Jordan. A vibrant Muslim community attracted her father to live his American life in Baltimore. Mr. Ali was a devout Muslim and lived a life of respect and dignity for all. He had come a long way since driving a taxi in Pakistan 40 years ago.

Ali opened a convenience store near the Orioles' home at Camden Yards. He wanted to be a sole owner and turned down generous offers from 7/11 and Circle K. One store became 2, and then 15. Her father reinvented himself as a supreme businessman, and yet, did not want to move from his original house. With all of his success, there was very little change in his material life. He did not want the community that he loved to think of him differently. There was no need for a façade, Mr. Ali remained true to himself within his Muslim community..

Olivia did not want to stray from her family and community. She completed her undergraduate work at the University of Alabama, medical School at Johns Hopkins. Her anesthesia residency and cardiothoracic fellowship were also at Johns Hopkins. She envisioned her life married with children. Olivia was particular. She would marry only a man from the community that she grew up in.

Olivia's focus was on medical education and developed teaching methods in the operating room that were light years ahead of the Socratic method. As a full professor, her research and writing were innovative techniques in education that overflowed from residency training to high schools.

Unlike her parents, Olivia and her husband, Muhammed, he did want material items. They renovated a modest home into an architectural masterpiece, with the outside of the house looking like any other in the community. The focus of the interior was the kitchen with the elite appliances and an island with eight chairs around it. This extravagance included five bedrooms, five bathrooms, a library, and a home entertainment theater. Her three children were raised as she had been, with an emphasis on a life of faith. While loyal to her Muslim community, she lived in a

C. Scher, *Anesthesia Conversations*,
https://doi.org/10.1007/978-3-032-05354-1_14

secular world outside of her community. She was able to compartmentalize her life inside and outside the community. She did not go to a mosque, followed a secular diet, and enjoyed an alcoholic drink.

A 17-year-old young boy presented to the emergency room with a chief complaint of being air hungry within moments after starting a soccer game. He had been the star in his league until extreme exhaustion set in 6 months ago at the 30-minute mark of a game. His exhaustion degenerated with minimal effort after a minute. Olivia had just intubated a 70-year-old with severe COPD. She was fascinated by the case in the next slot.

Olivia thought there were several essential questions that were not asked in the initial evaluation. With the help of a Creole interpreter, it was revealed that he was an illegal immigrant from Haiti. He had a brother who was 27 and a sister who was 15. He left Haiti 3 years ago and has not heard from his siblings since. He did remember that his father died at age 31. By word of mouth in the Haitian community, the consensus was that his mother was alive. He did remember that his older brother had become frail, soon before he left.

An EKG rhythm strip revealed a non-sustainable ventricular tachycardia. His chest x-ray demonstrated cardiomegaly. Blood was drawn for every lab test related to his heart. Olivia offered to do a transesophageal echocardiogram. It was two in the morning, and the cardiology team was tied up with the usual night of a line of patients with myocardial infarctions. With more than a struggle, a Creole interpreter was found but was unable to translate English medical jargon. There were no phone numbers in the chart, nor any documentation that the patient even existed. Olivia and the interventional cardiologist gave consent to two physicians. She planned to call one of the hospital social workers in the morning.

Olivia suggested that the case should be done in the morning. A full interventional cardiology team, pathologists, ultrasound-trained cardiologists, EP nurses, and the Biotronix company representative were all a must. The interventional fellow arranged that all of the essential staff would be available at 11 AM.

With all monitors placed, the patient was considered to be a "full stomach," and a rapid sequence induction of 14 mg of etomidate and 100 mg of succinylcholine was administered. His weight was 55 kilograms, and none of the markers of a difficult intubation made the passage of 8.0 endotracheal intubation easy. An EZ-cap and the anesthesia machine revealed carbon dioxide to confirm the tube was in the lungs. Olivia requested fluoroscopy to determine the distance between the endotracheal tube and the carina.

Nina and Olivia started the TEE examination. The four-chamber view was shocking. The cardiologist called for three attendings to see that the left ventricle was normal, but the right ventricle was almost akinetic. The echo revealed an ejection fraction of the left ventricle was 60% but the right ventricular ejection fraction was 7%. During the TEE, an EKG alarm revealed ventricular tachycardia at 130 beats per minute. 300 mg of Amiodarone normalized the heart rhythm to a normal sinus rhythm. The EP nursing team had put on the "shocking stickers" to convert almost any tachyarrhythmia.

"Have you not seen this before? It appears to be a classic case, by echo findings, of Arrhythmogenic Right Ventricular Cardiomyopathy" Nina was asking a question and boasting at the same time.

Olivia noted that there was a clot in the right ventricle. The low ejection fraction of the right ventricle was analogous to blood just sitting in the ventricle. The clot was a time bomb. Clots could enter the pulmonary vascular bed which could impede blood flow to the lungs. Blood that was deoxygenated would not be able to enter the lungs for oxygenation. The clot could become lodged in the brain!

An attending in cardiology went through the echo with his fellow. Olivia expressed her thoughts on what next should be done.

"The patient almost crashed after intubation. Let's wake him up and transport him to the cardiac ICU. We will form a team to collect all of the needed data under one anesthetic if possible. He will need an endomyocardial biopsy, an electrophysiologic study, insertion of an AICD and a Watchman. Long term anticoagulation in an unreliable teenager could lead to dangerous clots that could land systemically. The Watchman is inserted at the left atrial appendage and prevents clots from moving out of the heart to cause embolic strokes."

Olivia needed a social worker to hunt down his entire family. She read that the genetics of this disorder are autosomal dominant.

"By doing the math, it appears that the father died of it and the siblings certainly have it." went on. "Arrhythmogenic right ventricular cardiomyopathy is a fatty replacement of cardiac muscle in the right ventricle (ARVC). A patient may present with many dangerous arrhythmias so the defibrillator may only work for V-tach or V-fib. To my knowledge, there is no treatment of any benefit. I am not familiar with the transplant data on these cases but from what I see on my phone is that a heart transplant is the only choice for the kid to have a normal life."

"The anesthetic for the electrophysiologic study is complicated. The inhalational anesthetics are calcium channel blockers that will lower the ejection fraction. Any drug that is needed to raise the blood pressure, cannot simultaneously increase the pulmonary vascular resistance. Phenylephrine is a last choice. The anesthetic must be a total intravenous anesthetic." Olivia proceeded with dexmedetomidine, low-dose propofol, and low-dose remifentanil.

"The basic rules for an EP study are low tidal volumes (a jet ventilator would be ideal), minimal fluids (the field of study is showered with fluids that are absorbed) and the use of norepinephrine and vasopressin as needed. Phenylephrine will increase pulmonary vascular resistance which is problematic in an extremely low ejection fraction in the right ventricle. I want to give the lowest dose possible on each med. We need a BIS monitor for this case. If the EP team needs to induce an arrhythmia or pacing or intravenous isoproterenol. I would not induce with the usual drugs. I would just start the TIVA without boluses. When he is asleep, we can titrate remifentanil if need be.

I want to put in my own IV. I need at least 6 stopcocks attached to large bore IV. In many cases, I rarely do an awake arterial line but this case is clearly different. The risk and benefits have to be weighed carefully. The EP team needs femoral access for the study and the IJs for ICDs and other possible devices. I am good with one large bore or 2 with lesser bores."

Olivia scanned the literature, and a heart transplant is curative. UNOS (United Network Organ Sharing) was notified by the cardiologists. Due to frequent ventricular arrhythmias and RV predominant pathology, patients require unique considerations in regard to timing of evaluation, hemodynamic support options, and wait-listing qualifications.

The patient was placed near the top on the transplant list, and when his oxygen saturations hovered in the low eighties, the patient was placed on ECMO and heparin as a bridge to transplant. He passed on the second week of ECMO from a heparin-related intracranial hemorrhage.

Olivia was devastated and became the second victim. She played the "blame" game.

"The team reacted to poor choices rather than anticipate and treat preemptively. The speed to evaluate, initiation of anticoagulation, insertion of an ICD, ECMO and contacting UNOS took too long. The data on heart transplants was limited in the literature, based on a small cohort of cases. Contacting UNOS should have been done first. Every component of care, including UNOS contact and ECMO, should have been done on the first day."

"Due to the severity of his illness and young age, he would have been near the top of the transplant list in the UNOS District that they were in."

Olivia made these assumptions and could not understand that this was a patient in dire straits.

Olivia would view this to be a publishable UNOS case. The EP cardiologists defended themselves and reminded Olivia that UNOS was called on day one.

"The patient was on the top of the list" and "There was no heart available."

Olivia was pissed off and sad. The other members of the team thought that the care was excellent, but the patient was going to die despite their work.

Two hearts were offered to the patient from centers outside of their district. One was from New York and the other from Ohio. One heart was HIV+ and Hep C+.

Olivia lost it. "For fucks sake! Are you stupid! HIV and Hep. C are very treatable. First transplant, then treat the HEP C or HIV! There are case reports that despite immunosuppressant treatment for the new heart, this process remains successful!"

The cardiologist in charge, Dr. Kim blew a gasket. "Wrong Olivia. Immunosuppressant with HIV?

There are a few case reports and not all of them end well. Just Wrong!! The heart was rejected by many centers. Centers need good results and taking an HIV heart is not ideal. It could give the kid some more time, but he needed a pristine heart."

Olivia could not accept the level of ignorance. At a debriefing meeting after the death of the patient, her emotions took over, and she understood that immunosuppression and HIV were a tricky balance. Olivia cried out "I will never be part of another shit show that this team created. I am done!"

Olivia slammed the conference door shut and chose to walk up five flights to her office rather than take the elevator. With no one in the stairwell, she could cry in privacy and try to gather herself. Olivia arrived at her office and grabbed her purse, and left. She did not bother to change out of her scrubs and left her street clothes hanging over her office chair. Her phone was ringing, and if it was not her husband, she would not respond to the call. Olivia did not want to wait a minute to leave the hospital. She could see a United cab coming down Tulane Avenue and flagged it in time. She texted her husband, and he texted back that he just finished his case. He would have his fellow do all of the post-op work, and he would meet her at home ASAP.

Olivia, who calmed down in the cab, started to cry hysterically when John came home. He was able to piece sentences together from her hysteria. He suggested a leave of absence with no definitive return date. They did not need the money, and John wanted to wait until Olivia gathered herself.

John and Olivia plowed through a bottle of wine and ordered sushi for delivery. They talked for over an hour. John knew to validate her version and made a quick plan to fly up to New York City for R and R. They would see some shows, eat great food, and hit some museums.

While they had a great time, her anger level would go from zero to one hundred in seconds at the mention of the event. John suggested therapy, and surprisingly, Olivia was all in. While in New York, Olivia thought it was way too early to need a leave of absence. She claimed that she never had a mental health issue, and this would pass. John knew her well. Like most physicians and nurses, tragedy is part of professional life. They use whatever coping skills they have to move on to the next day and the next patient.

With one-on-one psychiatry, medications, and alternative medicine, there was little improvement. Her psychiatrist recommended group therapy, but there were no openings in the cognitive groups. There was a spot in the dialectical behavior group. After the first session, Olivia convinced herself that it was a waste of her time.

John was one of those with a gift of street smarts who thought that time would heal Olivia's state of mind. As time marched on, time did not change Olivia's mental status. John offered several solutions, all of which were met with a "No" before he was able to finish a sentence. He asked Olivia for 3 minutes without a disturbance.

"You have made a national name utilizing new techniques to teach medicine outside the classroom. Why not give up all clinical practice, or have cases that are simpler that allow you to keep teaching in the operating room. Another possibility is to aim high and follow the administrative path to become a Dean of a Medical School. My suggestion is to make a list of items in the case where you were successful and make a list of items that you think contributed to his death. Have a meeting with all of the providers of the case and hear their perspective." Within a month, John's most recent proposal did not work. He appeared to be clueless about psychiatry. Her psychiatrist's next suggestion was ECT. Olivia was so beaten down and agreed.

Suggested Reading

1. Gilljam T, Bergh. Right ventricular cardiomyopathy timing of heart transplantation in Uhi's anomaly and arrhythmogenic right ventricular cardiomyopathy. Eur J Heart Fail. 2009;11(1):106–9. https://doi.org/10.1093/eurjhf/hfn014. PMID: 19147464 Free article.
2. Khan S, Naz H, Khan MSQ, Ullah A, Satti DI, Malik J, Mehmoodi A. The WATCHMAN device review: a new era for stroke prophylaxis. J Community Hosp Intern Med Perspect. 2023;13(3):10–20. https://doi.org/10.55729/2000-9666.1183. eCollection 2023. PMID: 37877058.
3. Maitra NS, Dugger SJ, Balachandran IC, Civitello AB, Khazanie P, Rogers JG. Impact of the 2018 UNOS heart transplant policy changes on patient outcomes. JACC Heart Fail. 2023;11(5):491–503. https://doi.org/10.1016/j.jchf.2023.01.009. Epub 2023 Mar 1. PMID: 36892486 Review.
4. Patel H, Shah P, Patel P, Rampal U, Shamoon F, Tiyyagura S. Arrhythmogenic right ARVD/C and catecholaminergic polymorphic ventricular tachycardia (CPVT): a phenotypic spectrum seen in the same patient. 2015;48(5):874–8. https://doi.org/10.1016/j.jelectrocard.2015.06.005. Epub 2015 Jun 7. PMID: 26082335.
5. Zens T, Ochoa B, Eldredge RS, Molitor M. Pediatric venoarterial and venovenous. ECMO Semin Pediatr Surg. 2023;32(4):151327. https://doi.org/10.1016/j.sempedsurg.2023.151327. Epub 2023 Oct 27. PMID: 37956593.

Modes of Ventilation in Premature Babies in Respiratory Distress

15

Lucy Benetez

There were never enough challenges in Lucy's life. The challenges could be in medicine and in her world outside of medicine. She was born in San Juan, Puerto Rico, and was 5 years out of her residency. Her undergraduate, medical school, residency, and fellowship in pediatric anesthesia were all at the University of Miami.

Her parents came to the United States in the sixties and took a similar route at The University of Miami for all of their education. Lucy's father was the baseball coach at the University of Miami, and her mother was a Professor of Law and a federal prosecutor in Dade County. Her parents defined the word "driven," which put Lucy on a crash course on multi-tasking in her life and "burnout". Times of burnout affected her for only brief times in her life. She never had the insight to know what was going on inside her brain.

There are hundreds of pediatric anesthesiologists in the country, and she wanted a niche in the field that was consistent with her clinical and research goals. During her pediatric anesthesia fellowship, she wanted to spend as much time as possible in the neonatal (NICU). The ACGME approved her time in her fellowship in the NICU. This unique request was not unconditional. Lucille had to keep a log of all the hours spent in the NICU and the procedures done and send them back to the ACGME weekly.

Lucy was intense in her work and a touch less in her personal life. She was a very attractive woman, but most dates went nowhere as men found her too "intense and self-centered." Her dating failure gave her enough insight to seek a therapist.

After 6 months of psychotherapeutics, she improved. She was able to "bring the temperature down" that allowed her to start and maintain relationships. As she would only have it, she had a steady relationship with a pediatric surgeon who was 5 years her senior. He, like her, was in therapy for thinking "he was right all the time." Six months into their relationship, they were engaged and the wedding would include almost 300 people. Both families were huge. The running joke is that newlyweds would go to the Arctic Circle to study climate change rather than go to Paris or a Four Seasons in Hawaii and chill by the beach.

C. Scher, *Anesthesia Conversations*,
https://doi.org/10.1007/978-3-032-05354-1_15

Lucille was surprised to see several premature babies born at less than 28 weeks of gestation and survive. She was next up for the next NICU admission. Lucille was not required to do any night calls, but once a weekday, she would stay 24 hours. There was no night or day in the NICU, and the 24-hour cycle included so many more patients and patient complications during the night. She was aware that with modern NICU medicine, infant mortality declined but severe complications had not changed other than bronchopulmonary dysplasia (BPD).

The accepted current etiology of BPD, surrounded inflammation in premature lungs. These neonates need respiratory support and the mode of ventilation could be a "game changer." The literature suggests that noninvasive ventilation lowers the incidence of lung disease compared to endotracheal mechanical ventilation.

A mother at 28 weeks of gestation went into labor at her home, 80 miles from a hospital. Her neonate was born in the bathroom. Like most of the severely premature children, the baby could survive but not escape the horrific comorbidities. Intraventricular hemorrhage and BPD were the rule rather than the exception.

Respiratory distress presents only minutes after birth with a grunting sound that is a neonate's attempt at endogenous CPAP. Lucille intubated the neonate, as soon as she arrived in the Neonatal ICU. After intubation, Lucy gave two trials of Exosurf (surfactant) followed by extubation. In the severely premature baby, surfactant was not the only pulmonary deficiency. Many lungs are hypoplastic. The alveoli and blood vessels are "too far apart to allow oxygen to make the transition from alveoli to the bloodstream." As expected, the required ventilatory support and umbilical line placement. The baby was extubated and transitioned to noninvasive ventilation.

There are five modes of noninvasive ventilation that are used worldwide. Lucille had to choose the mode of ventilation that matched the clinical picture of the neonate and the resources of the hospital. She was a firm believer that noninvasive respiratory pressure was superior to the "old school" intubation and mechanical ventilation.

The NICU pediatric faculty chose HFNC (High Flow Nasal Cannula) for their patients. The benefits of HFNC include achievement of a more stable FIO2 at a higher flow rate, a reduction of dead space, and a reduction of air resistance from warm and humidified air. HFNC is associated with a modest decrease in respiratory rate and a decrease in minute volume with improved oxygen saturation without alteration in tidal volume.

The second choice was a possibility, but Lucy ruled it out. Oscillation by comparison has a limited temperature range, poor thermal stability, and low accuracy. One of the primary goals of nasal ventilation was to get the most absorbable calories in without accruing all of the comorbidities that were potentially in front of him. Lucille took all of the credit for choosing the baby's lung protection by not having BPD or a pneumothorax. The elemental feeds were perfect. The baby's weight gain was remarkable. The baby developed a grade 2 intraventricular bleed. Only time would tell if there were any significant neurological sequelae from the bleed.

Lucy's husband knew when to keep his distance when Lucille was wrapped up in the intensity of this case. Lucille blamed herself for the intraventricular bleed, which was preposterous since the dynamics of the intraventricular bleed are not well known. It was believed that the lack of autoregulation in the germinal matrix was causal. It was surmised that hypertension might have affected the integrity of the germinal matrix of the vessels (vessels along the ventriculus that have little support). There is a very fine line between the integrity of the "doctor's credit," in spite of "everything that could be done was done" versus pure iatrogenesis. For the rest of her clinical life, Lucille felt strongly that every bad outcome was due to provider error. That was Lucy, just being Lucy.

After 2 years of total immersion with all of her patients, Lucille's husband thought that Lucille had only two options: to do a three-year full residency in pediatrics or simply stop taking care of NICU and return to the OR full time. A second residency would be more than exhausting. Lucille's husband was relieved that she took a step back and went back to giving anesthesia full time.

Lucille's intensity did not wane. Her tempered enthusiasm was back to the pedal on the metal. Her husband grew weary of her intensity and came home one evening and told her that her work was having a strong negative impact on him. Lucille was speechless. While he was packing to leave her, she was busy reading an anesthesia journal as if nothing had happened. She buried her emotions and her total appearance of cool, calm, and collected which was exactly how she felt.

After multiple attempts by her husband for reconciliation, she remained "cold," and after 6 months, she agreed to sign the divorce papers given to her. It was a simple divorce: no children, no money issues, and no abuse.

Lucille never married again. She went back and did a three-year pediatric residency and became a member of the NICU faculty. Her husband remarried 18 months after the divorce. Lucille went on to have over 60 peer-reviewed papers, multiple textbooks, and became an invited speaker all over the world. Lucille knew that a family with children would block the successful woman that she had become. Over the years, she had three or four relationships that failed for the same problem. She was aware of her intensity that kept men away. She did not want to change her intensity.

Chris met Lucy on the Starbucks line at the American Society of Anesthesiology Annual Meeting in San Francisco. He had been tracking her career and was feeling desperate. He did not think he could give her a faculty position to match the soaring career path she insisted on being on. He invited her to travel to the Crescent City and give Grand Rounds on whatever topic she picked, Chris would fly her down, put her up at the Ritz-Carlton, take her for dinner at Revolution, and have breakfast with the residents at the Ritz.

"Wow! Your department must have beaucoup bucks"

"No, I do."

She walked back to her hotel after dinner. She called Chris to let him know that she was all in.

Chris did not give her an administrative role. He just wanted her to continue in her best mode, free to do as she pleased.

Suggested Reading

1. Chen IL, Chen HL. New developments in neonatal respiratory management. Pediatr Neonatol. 2022;63(4):341–7. https://doi.org/10.1016/j.pedneo.2022.02.002. Epub 2022 Mar 16. PMID: 35382987.
2. Deger J, Goethe EA, LoPresti MA, Lam S. Intraventricular hemorrhage in premature infants: a historical review. World Neurosurg. 2021;153:21–5. https://doi.org/10.1016/j.wneu.2021.06.043. Epub 2021 Jun 16.
3. Gilfillan M, Bhandari A, Bhandari V. Diagnosis and management of bronchopulmonary dysplasia. BMJ. 2021;375:n1974. https://doi.org/10.1136/bmj.n1974. PMID: 34670756 Review.
4. Ramaswamy VV, More K, Roehr CC, Bandiya P, Nangia S. Efficacy of noninvasive respiratory support modes for primary respiratory distress syndrome: systemic review and network meta-analysis. Pediatr Pulmonol. 2020;55(11):2940–63. https://doi.org/10.1002/ppul.25011. Epub 2020 Sept 4. PMID: 32762014.
5. Schulzke SM, Stoecklin B. Update on ventilatory management of the extremely preterm infants- Neonatal Intensive Care Unit perspective. Paediatr Anaesth. 2022;32(2):363–71. https://doi.org/10.1111/pan.14369. Epub 2021 Dec 15. PMID: 34878697.

16 Severe Pulmonary Hypertension in the Pregnant Patient

Susan Mullins

Susan's obstetrician, Tom Porto. consulted the cardiology team after Susan's prenatal visit. She had never been pregnant, and she attributed her difficulty breathing and severe fatigue to pregnancy. Dr. Schiff, Chair of the Department of Cardiology, was more than concerned when she entered the office. Susan was 15 weeks pregnant and described dyspnea with just getting out of the car. Susan had dyspnea before she was pregnant that was noticeable 6 months before she conceived. Her 14 hours of sleep each night was almost shocking for someone who was an anesthesiologist getting 5–6 hours of sleep. Her husband knew that there was something very wrong.

Dr. Porto put in an order for an ultrasound of the fetus. All was well with the ultrasound. The baby's size was appropriate for gestational age. The quantity of the amniotic fluid was perfect. The fetal heartbeat was normal. All of the major organs were visualized and appeared healthy. While early in gestation, the anatomy of the fetus was excellent. Susan's pulse oximeter read 90%, which was of severe concern. He called for a cardiac consultation for Susan.

Cardiology arrived 30 minutes after the consultation was requested. It could be weeks before your appointment for an echocardiogram, but this was a true STAT. Susan and her husband Ted were escorted to the ECHO lab. The tech performed the ECHO in 20 minutes. The only one who receives the results is the cardiologist. Susan and Ted returned to Dr. Schiff's conference room, and every seat around the conference table was taken except the seats for Susan, Ted, and Dr. Goldberg. Dr. Ari Goldberg, Clinical Director of the Pulmonary Hypertension Research Unit, started the conversation.

"Susan, you have pulmonary hypertension. It probably started years before you became pregnant. Similarly to systemic high blood pressure, the blood pressure in your lung vessels is very high. The pulmonary arterial vessels are so constricted that blood in the right ventricle cannot pump blood into the lungs for oxygenation. Women with pulmonary hypertension have a high risk of morbidity and mortality during pregnancy. The inability to increase cardiac output leads to heart failure while further risks are introduced with hypercoagulability and decrease in systemic

C. Scher, *Anesthesia Conversations*,
https://doi.org/10.1007/978-3-032-05354-1_16

vascular resistance. Pregnancy was regarded as a contraindication in women with pulmonary hypertension.

I would like you to have pulmonary artery catheterization to measure specifically the range of blood pressures in your lungs. That will determine how your right ventricle will hold up with changes in pulmonary artery pressure."

Sussan did not need this presentation of pulmonary hypertension. She was the senior member of the obstetrical anesthesia section. While she gave this presentation at Trinity many times herself, her perspective on this discussion was frightening, and she wondered how many women must have been frightened by her own presentation. She was surprised that the presentation was dumbed down for her, while she thought that more science was needed in Dr. Goldberg's explanation.

"Pulmonary hypertension is defined as an increase in mean pulmonary arterial pressure (mPAP) ≥25 mmHg at rest. The histopathology includes medial hypertrophy, intimal proliferation, fibrosis, thrombotic lesions and venous thickening. Many pathways are involved in the abnormal proliferation and contraction of the smooth muscle cells of the pulmonary arteries in patients with pulmonary arterial hypertension. Three of these pathways are important since they have been targeted with drugs that are endothelin receptor antagonists, phosphodiesterase type 5 (PDE-5) inhibitors and prostacyclin derivatives."

Susan was sensing that termination at 19 weeks would be the cardiologist's recommendation. As a devout Catholic, Susan faced one of the most painful dilemmas in a woman's life. Her faith would help her to have a healthy baby, and God would keep her safe. Susan felt blessed with motherhood.

Susan had a long talk with her husband Ted, who already had his own take on the event. Ted was freaking out. He started to sweat which was his usual response to utter fear. He was writing down on a piece of newspaper questions that were rapidly firing in his brain. He would let Dr. Goldberg finish his dissertation. By the time he was finished, most of his questions he wrote in the newspaper were addressed.

"During labor and delivery, the risk of complications builds on each other. Labor and delivery increase PA pressure due to volume shifts resulting from blood loss and uterine contractions, vasovagal reaction to pain, acidosis, and hypercarbia, leading to a further increase in pulmonary vascular resistance and an increased risk of thromboembolic complications. I am not exaggerating when I say the incidence of death is high, near 50%. I tell patients not to become pregnant or abort. If you are determined to deliver, then our team of experts, including obstetrics and anesthesiology, will be challenged to the highest level possible. Everything that can be done will be done to have an excellent outcome". Dr. Porto sounded conflicted. He was.

Susan was forty and feeling that this was her last chance to have a baby. She chose not to abort. Dr. Porto suggested that Susan and Ted be alone to discuss the entire event. The presentation was crystal clear. They stood by their decision, and Susan said, "bring it on".

Susan decided to accept the odds of carrying the baby to birth, but she needed to know the PA pressure. Susan had a PA pressure of 70 mmHg systolic as measured by right heart catheterization. The efficacy of medications is reduced at this level not significantly, she was followed weekly, and the PA pressure measured by echocardiography was consistently 65. Dr. Goldberg felt that 60 could become 80. If a spinal or epidural anesthetic needed to be converted to a general anesthetic, hemorrhage, nausea, and vomiting could increase the pulmonary artery pressure to a life-threatening event.

Susan was admitted to the hospital at 36 weeks for endothelin receptor agonists, among other medications. At the beginning of her 37th week, Susan went into full labor. She was given a subcutaneous injection of terbutaline, and the labor stopped. She was in labor for only 10 minutes and could not catch her breath. Dr. Porto mobilized his team for a STAT C-section with a combined spinal/epidural. The baby was born healthy, and Susan was never not air hungry during the case.

Dr. Goldberg stopped by Susan's room the morning after delivery. The topic of discussion was listing Susan for transplanted lungs. The five-year survival rate was 87%. Susan was all in. The United Network Sharing organization was notified, and Susan was placed high on the transplant list.

She moved up to the waiting list quickly as her situation had become clinically dire. With her death imminent, her lungs became available for transplantation. After two stormy months, Susan was well and worked her way back to being an anesthesiologist again.

Suggested Reading

1. Arial SR, Moussa H, Sinkey R, Dhungana R, Tallaj JA, Pamboukian SV, Patarroyo-Aponte M, Acharya D, Bajaj NS, Bhattarai S, Lenneman A, Joly JM, Sibai BM. Management of reproductive health in patients with pulmonary hypertension. Am J Obstet Gynecol MFM. 2020;2(2):100087. https://doi.org/10.1016/j.ajogmf.2020.100087. Epub 2020 Jan 23. PMID: 33345958 Review.
2. Barańska-Pawełczak K, Wojciechowska C, Jacheć W. Pregnancy in patients with pulmonary arterial hypertension in light of the new ESC guidelines on pulmonary hypertension. Int J Environ Res Public Health. 2023;20(5):4625. https://doi.org/10.3390/ijerph20054625. PMID: 36901635 Review.
3. Bos S, Vos R, Van Raemdonck DE, Verleden GM. Survival in adult lung transplantation: where are we in 2020. Curr Opin Organ Transplant. 2020;25(3):268–73. https://doi.org/10.1097/MOT.0000000000000753. PMID: 32332197.
4. Mészáros M, Bikov A. The nitric oxide pathway in pulmonary arterial hypertension: pathomechanism biomarkers and drug targets. Curr Med Chem. 2020;27(42):7168–88. https://doi.org/10.2174/0929867327666200522215047. PMID: 32442078.
5. Quinn JF, Whittaker MR, Davis TP. Delivering nitric oxide with nanoparticles. J Control Release. 2015;205:190–205. https://doi.org/10.1016/j.jconrel.2015.02.007. Epub 2015 Feb PMID: 256658655.
6. Singh I, Horn E, Haythe J. Pulmonary hypertension in pregnancy. Clin Chest Med. 2021;42(1):91–9. https://doi.org/10.1016/j.ccm.2020.10.006. Epub 2021 Jan 9. PMID: 33541621 Review.

Anesthesia for Obstetrical Hemorrhage 17

Andrew Phillips, Juliana Wilson, Lily Xuan

Amy and Andrew were on the same obstetrical floor at the UT Southwestern Hospital in Dallas, Texas. Amy was one of three Chief Residents in the largest obstetrical residency training program in the United States. There were 18 new residents every year. Amy's exposure to high-risk pregnancies covered every conceivable obstetrical board question, from her training at Parkland and Clements University Hospital.

Andrew completed his anesthesia residency at the University of Iowa and obstetrical anesthesia fellowship at UT Southwestern. He became an attending obstetrical anesthesiologist and after 2 years, he was promoted to Chief of Obstetrical Anesthesia at UT Southwestern. He spearheaded the endeavor of having a seven-bed Obstetrical Intensive Care Unit and recruited two attendings who were board certified in critical care.

Andrew admired Amy's intense immersion in the care of her patients. She was a bit of a pain in the ass. She insisted on her own care in the new intensive care unit. Amy also operated on gyn-oncology cases, a surgical field in which she had no formal training. She was relentless on the demands she put on the obstetrical anesthesia team. The Chair of Obstetrics had to put up with her questionable professional manners. She was the leading biller at the four hospitals that were part of the department. Nothing more to say.

Amy finally took some time off. She had a strong family and only professional friends. She went alone to Jazz Fest and became hooked. The Chair of Obstetrics was more than happy to write letters for Amy. She was out of his hair and on the way to New Orleans. As they were becoming more than friends, Andrew went with her.

In the 5 years that she was in a solo practice in Metairie, Louisiana. She alone amassed the most patients than any group practice in Jefferson Parish. She was not an OB-GYN but just an OB. Her practice evolved into 7 days a week, 24 hours a day. To give her time to rest, she followed the plan of "the 5:00 PM" C-section; a practice just to clear the board to fit in something to eat and hopefully a few hours of sleep. Amy had not home cooked a meal in years, and her parents "had to

C. Scher, *Anesthesia Conversations*,
https://doi.org/10.1007/978-3-032-05354-1_17

convince her" to come home to LA. They were concerned about her physical and mental health. Amy lived in scrubs, gave up on makeup, exercise, and her nutrition. She was 100 pounds, down from 130.

The time had arrived for the search for partners. She had to get some balance in her life. Her offer to new hires was exceptional. The hirees had to be young women, and Amy would start by splitting all the money earned equally three ways. This highly unusual arrangement did incentivize Cara and Cynthia to become partners. As CEO, Amy could add patients from other hospitals. While Amy wanted to slow down, her reputation was that she would never slow down.

Cara and Cynthia thought they hit the jackpot. Cara trained at Texas Tech, and Cynthia trained at Northwestern. At first, they could not believe that Amy was able to hold it together by covering three hospitals by herself. They worked harder than they could have imagined, but the three of them bonded at the highest professional level.

The only demand that challenged their own training was to adopt Amy's manner of clinical practice. (1) No epidurals before the patient had less than 4 cm of dilation. (2) Discuss all cases with the blood bank. Blood needed to be available for every one of their patients. (3) Epidural catheters would be pulled as soon as the case was over, leaving lesser modalities to treat post-C-section pain. (4) No parents in the OR for C-sections and (5) Patients must be able to push and have a painless delivery. Amy always had "issues" with the obstetrical anesthesiologists. She always undervalued her anesthesia colleagues. Andrews was concerned that he could not keep up with her.

Amy's exhaustion, mood, nutrition, chaotic sleep, and isolation, made her life was of control. Cara and Cynthia knew that they were not there to make life easier for Amy. Amy would just look for more work. As CEO of her group of three, she could explore future hospital affiliations, entertain possible buyouts by large healthcare networks, and determine whether to accept or deny the health insurance of the patients. After 1 year, the other hirees would be able to participate in these decisions and all of the power that Amy had. Above all, Amy would always keep the hirees abreast of all endeavors that passed her way.

The estimated blood loss associated with a normal vaginal delivery is 500 cc and 1000 cc for a C-section.

The anesthesiologist viewed that anyone could have one or many risk factors for uterine atony and hemorrhage. Above all, the blood bank was able to organize a system of blood delivery to keep up with Amy's fear of severe uterine hemorrhage.

The causes of postpartum hemorrhage can be summarized by the four "T's": tone (uterine atony), trauma (lacerations or uterine rupture), tissue (retained placenta or clots), and thrombin (clotting-factor deficiency) The most common cause is uterine atony (accounting for approximately 70% of cases), followed by obstetric lacerations (approximately 20%), retained placental tissue (approximately 10%), and clotting-factor deficiencies (<1%).

A 22-year-old G1P0 presented to the high-risk obstetrical service for an assessment of the likelihood of postpartum hemorrhage. The patient's medical history as related to uterine hemorrhage included: (1) type 1 diabetes, (2) pregnancy-induced hypertension, (3) family history of uterine hypotonia, and (4) being an underserved patient. Andrew did not want an epidural or spinal for high-risk patients.

Andrew did not want to impose a sympathectomy in a possible case of uterine hemorrhage.

The baby was born 10 minutes after the initial incision. Pitocin was administered as in all cases of the beginning of uterine atony, methergine and hemabate follow. The uterus remained atonic despite external massage and the uterotonics. At no time was there a visible clot.

Andrew called for help, and Lily and Juliana were there within 5 minutes. Both agreed to activate the massive transfusion protocol. Juliana placed a 14-gauge IV in the right antecubital fossa. The Belmont rapid infuser was brought to the OR by anesthesia tech. PRBCs and FFP went into the reservoir, and products entered the 14-gauge IV. Platelets and cryo transfused directly to the in situ 18-gauge.

Lily screamed "TXA" STAT!!. Andrew strongly suggested that Von Willebrand's could be the cause of the coagulopathy.

Amy had been down the road of uterine atony over 100 times. Amy lost her cool when Andrew mentioned Von Willerbrands. Her plan was a balloon in the uterus. "Just keep up with blood products or pressers or whatever you normally do for atony" I know my patients well. This woman does not have von Willebrand's.

Andrew ignored Amy and started the process to treat von Willebrand's disease. The signs and symptoms of the disease are highly variable, and this patient's only symptom was heavy menstrual periods.

von Willebrand factor (VWF) is a large adhesive glycoprotein required for platelet adhesion to the subendothelium at the site of vessel injury, platelet aggregation to form a platelet plug, and stabilization of factor 8 in the circulation. The explanation for how an autoimmune disease causes von Willebrand disease is in the activation of von Willebrand factor proteins.

In many cases of acquired von Willebrand disease, the von Willebrand factor protein has an abnormal clearance level. Enhanced or elevated clearance levels of the von Willebrand factor lead to the development of the inherited Type 1 variety of von Willebrand's disease. Factor 8 and VWF have been linked to each other. The way that Amy thinks about it is by drawing the number 8. The top half of the eight is factor 8 and the bottom of the eight is VWF.

Many autoimmune diseases coexist with other autoimmune diseases. Acquired von Willebrand disease has been linked to a number of triggers: (1) Lupus (2) Scleroderma (3) Antiphospholipid antibody syndrome, and (4) Hypothyroidism. Acquired forms of this disease can often be resolved by treating the underlying cause. Desmopressin causes endothelial cells to release von Willebrand factor into the bloodstream to be effective in clot formation.

Lily wanted to be prepared in case Andrew was right. If it were Von Willebrand's, there was no harm in treatment. She took her phone out to determine the intravenous dose of desmopressin in adults; 0.3 mcg/kg/dose (Max: 20 mcg/dose) IV once. The need for repeat dosage based on laboratory response and patient's clinical condition. A repeat dose after 8 to 12 hours and once daily thereafter as needed to reduce spontaneous or traumatic bleeding. Tachyphylaxis may occur with repeated administration given more frequently than once every 48 hours. The initial response is reproducible if desmopressin is given every 2 to 3 days.

Desmopressin helped a clot to form, and a fibrinolytic drug (TXA) made the clot stable. The amount of blood products administered slowed down. The uterus was saved in this young woman, and unused blood was sent back to the blood bank. Amy and Juliana did what so many physicians do now: get data off their cell phones. With TXA and Desmopressin administered, there was a visible clot in the field. Intrauterine balloons were inflated for 24 hours, and the uterus was saved.

Suggested Reading

1. Bos S, Vos R, Van Raemdonck DE, Verleden GM. Survival in adult lung transplantation: where are we in 2020? Curr Opin Organ Transplant. 2020;25(3):268–73. https://doi.org/10.1097/MOT.0000000000000753. PMID: 32332197.
2. Castaman G, James PD. Pregnancy and delivery in women with von Willebrand disease. Eur J Haematol. 2019;103(2):73–9. https://doi.org/10.1111/ejh.13250. Epub 2019 May 31. PMID: 31107984 Review.
3. Kotloff RM, Thabut G. Lung transplantation. Am J Respir Crit Care Med. 2011;184(2):159–71. https://doi.org/10.1164/rccm.201101-0134CI. Epub 2011 Mar 31.
4. Muñoz M, Stensballe J, Ducloy-Bouthors AS, Bonnet MP, De Robertis E, Fornet I, Goffinet F, Hofer S, Holzgreve W, Manrique S, Nizard J, Christory F, Samama CM, Hardy JF. Patient blood management in obstetrics: prevention and treatment of postpartum hemorrhage. A NATA consensus statement. Blood Transfus. 2019;17(2):112–36. https://doi.org/10.2450/2019.0245-18. Epub 2019 Feb 6. PMID: 30865585.
5. Post SE, Rood KM, Kiefer MK. Interventions of Postpartum Hemorrhage. Obstet Gynecol. 2023;66(2):367–83. https://doi.org/10.1097/GRF.0000000000000785. Epub 2023 May 5. PMID: 37204172.

18 Rona Hapern: An Anesthesiologist Who Was a Drug Addict, Broke, Pregnant, and an Oncology Case

Rona Hapern, William Robinson

Rona Halpern had been practicing anesthesia for 10 years. She never married. She had relationship issues and had been in therapy for the last 2 years. With no family, she should have accumulated enough money to be financially comfortable. William Robinson was her best friend on the faculty and was blown away when she asked him for a loan of 100,000 dollars. Rona was broke. She claimed to have invested poorly, and her cash flow was low from her addiction.

William, in his perfect friend mode, asked no questions and agreed to write her a check. The check did not have any impact on his financial status and recommended the financial advisor whom he worked with.

"It is five o'clock. Time for Happy Hour!" Rona's condo would have made it to "Architectural Digest." She essentially tore the condo down, each room down to the studs. The kitchen had the most expensive and functional appliances, and each bedroom was fitted with California closets. There was a heated swimming pool out back. The theme of the decor was super modern French and Italian walls and furniture. The air conditioner could cool down the SuperDome.

William made two pristine vodka martinis, and they were both ready for a second one 10 minutes after the first martinis were finished. The goal here was simple. Rona said it loud and clear, "let's get wasted!' William planned to dig deeper into the loan when Rona juggled between being clear-headed and totally drunk.

"I have not been able to save. My cocaine, weed, alcohol and heroin are expensive. I lost my sobriety during residency. I believe I have developed do or die skills on hiding hints. This has been going on for years! Did you have a single clue I was doing this?"

William was simply shocked! I had no idea. "Is the money needed solely to buy drugs?"

"It is money that I owe in this cycle of buying and using The threats to my fucked up life are becoming a reality. I have never even considered sobriety as the burden of not using is worse than the fear of using. There is a second big ticket item."

C. Scher, *Anesthesia Conversations*,
https://doi.org/10.1007/978-3-032-05354-1_18

"I am 15 weeks pregnant! I am so fucked up, I was at a party and was so wasted, I have no idea who the father is! I feel the noose around my neck. I have hidden my life from you, my family and friends. I do not think anyone believes I have a problem. You are the only one who knows I am pregnant."

"William transitioned by being a little buzzed to sensible and analytical. While William was a recovering addict from valium, he never took any drugs including weed."

"Cocaine use during pregnancy is associated with maternal migraines, seizures, premature membrane rupture, and separation of the placental lining from the uterus prior to delivery. Pregnancy is accompanied by normal cardiovascular changes, and cocaine use exacerbates these—sometimes leading to serious problems with high blood pressure, spontaneous miscarriage, preterm labor, and difficult delivery.

It is difficult to estimate the full extent of the consequences of maternal drug use and to determine the specific hazard of a particular drug to the unborn child, such as the amount and number of all drugs used, including nicotine or alcohol. Prenatal care; socioeconomic conditions; maternal nutrition; other health conditions, can all interact to influence maternal child outcomes. The baby will be withdrawing shortly after delivery.

Neonatal abstinence syndrome (NAS) refers to the fact that a newborn is a "drug addict." NAS happens when a baby gets addicted to a drug before birth and then goes through drug withdrawal after birth. Symptoms usually begin shortly after birth and can last several weeks. Symptoms of NAS include tremors, increased irritability, trouble sleeping, and excessive crying. It takes longer for a developing baby or newborn to get cocaine out of their system than it does an adult."

Something bothered Rona. Will seemed to know specifics about addiction and pregnancy.

Babies born to mothers who use cocaine during pregnancy are often prematurely delivered, have low birth weights, smaller head circumferences, and are shorter in length than babies born to mothers who do not use cocaine. The fact that most of these children do not show serious overt deficits should not be overinterpreted to indicate that there is no cause for concern.

Scientists are now finding that exposure to cocaine during fetal development may lead to subtle, yet significant, later deficits in some children. These include behavior problems and deficits in some aspects of cognitive performance, information processing, and sustained attention to tasks; abilities that are important for the realization of a child's full potential. Some deficits persist into the later years, with prenatally exposed adolescents showing increased risk for subtle problems with language and memory. Brain scans in teens suggest that at rest, the functioning of some brain regions, including areas involved in attention, planning, and language, may differ from that of nonexposed peers.

"There are at least 3 different intertwined problems; your addiction, your pregnancy and your job. You will not give anesthesia while you anesthetize yourself. It's difficult to estimate the full extent of the consequences of maternal drug use and to determine the specific hazard of a particular drug, such as the amount and number of all drugs used, including nicotine or alcohol. Prenatal care, socioeconomic conditions, maternal nutrition and other health conditions, can all interact to influence maternal child outcomes.

The baby will be born as an addict and enter the world as an addict." William googled pregnancy and addiction. It was painful to read. Advice would not be possible without the exhaustive research he usually does when his knowledge on a medical problem is on unsteady ground. He found NAS.

William picked up that exposure to cocaine during fetal development may lead to significant deficits in some children. "These include behavior problems and deficits in cognitive performance, information processing, and sustained attention to tasks. These abilities are important for a child's full potential. Some deficits persist into the later years, with prenatally exposed adolescents showing increased risk for subtle problems with language and memory."

Rona was distracted during Williams's comments on what lies in front of both Rona and the baby. Rona was focused on the challenges of her next fix. She was shivering and sweating at the same time. Rona complained of severe nausea and started wretching.

"Rona, it is time to go to the hospital. If William had left, she would have taken the 100K and bought drugs. Rona resisted at first but knew that her life was totally fucked. She showered, put on some jeans, a Nike tee shirt and flip-flops and entered the front passenger side of William's Beamer. Her only luggage was a large backpack."

After a two-hour drive, William stopped at the circular driveway of the "Fairway"; a "lavish" psychiatric hospital on 30 acres of New England's finest residential property. William called Fairway yesterday and asked what Rona was to pack: toiletries, jeans for four nights, tee shirts for a week, shoes without laces, no belts, and no pants that had to be tied. Essentially, she stripped down to the bones and no items that could result in a suicide. Cell phones were prohibited, and each resident was allowed to make one daily telephone call from Fairway's land line which was in each unit.

Rona was under the care of a team that included a social worker, a physician boarded in internal medicine, an addiction psychologist, and a psychiatrist. An obstetrical evaluation was of immediate concern, and an appointment was made on Rona's second day at Fairway.

The addiction plan was 2 weeks in lockdown followed by on-campus housing for 1 month. Rona's next step was a supervised job off-campus. The last 2 months were completely outpatient with daily drug tests and 5 meetings a week. This generic recovery plan was individualized based on each patient's other psychiatric and medical diagnoses. Front and center for Rona was the plan for her baby. Cell phones were prohibited and each resident was allowed to make a telephone call from Fairway's land line which was the sole phone in each unit.

Rona was severely depressed and was consumed, every day while in lockdown, with 10 different ways on how she would get drugs into the center. Her brain and her body were severely damaged. A supervised taper would start on day one. The success of the taper depended on what drugs she confessed to Rona had fear of withdrawal symptoms and fear of the future.

Lockdown is Lockdown. No matter how luxurious the hospital is. Lockdown at Fairway had no differences than any other lockdown. There were no doors or closets. Going to the bathroom was not a private affair. The floors were concrete with plastic on top to facilitate mopping with a bleach-based cleanser. Other than a bed, there was no furniture. There was a toilet but no shower. The door locked from the outside, and there was no way out. Bed checks were done every hour and the food served was meticulously prepared in the Mediterranean style.

There was a mandatory hour in the gym which had the most modern workout machines and a four-lane lap pool. There was clear scientific evidence that proved that daily aerobic exercise could reduce the fatty buildup in the liver in the alcoholic addicted patient. It was conclusive that most drugs impaired brain function and brain structure. The pool could reverse some significant cognitive loss. Rona chose the pool rather than running around an indoor track.

William was her health care proxy, and Rona gave permission for William to view all of her tests and results. He was relieved that she was HIV and Hep C negative. Her ESR and C-reactive protein levels were 3 times normal. The red cells were microcytic, and her platelet count was 500,000. The creatinine and liver function tests were normal. On the physical exam, there was widespread lymphadenopathy. Her medical tests and abnormal physical exam moved to front and center.

The issues were mounting. The psychiatrists were reluctant for her to withdraw from her addiction before an evaluation of laboratory results. and a physical exam. Dr. Trevor David was an oncologist who was referred to by one of the psychiatrists. His full evaluation was based on a bone marrow aspirate, bone marrow biopsy, lymph node biopsy, and blood smear. The results were consistent with Non-Hodgkin's Lymphoma.

By dates, Rona was in her first semester, the peak time of organogenesis. Dr. David strongly favored termination as treatment. Lymphoma treatment of the pregnant patient in the first semester consisted of chemotherapy and possible radiation. Chemotherapy is devastating for fetal well-being. An ultrasound of the fetus was consistent with a gestation of 14 weeks. Rona was conflicted about having a baby. This was her way out.

Rona asked William to be the anesthesiologist for the termination. He did not believe Rona had a full stomach. During his time as an attending, the full stomach in the pregnant patient began,\ at a very conservative 15 weeks. Over time, anesthesiologists believed that a full stomach began at 20 weeks. General anesthesia with intubation was the best choice for anesthesia; the pregnant patient was considered to have a full stomach at 20 weeks. William made it simple and chose sedation.

After 2 hours in the recovery room, Rona was transported back to the Fairway lockdown unit to deal with her severe dysphoria of a "supervised detox." There was quite a recipe of drugs in her body, each with a particular withdrawal time. The benzos could take months of sleeplessness and a wide array of symptoms; pervasive nausea, muscle cramps, tinnitus, and auditory hallucinations. She claimed to hear a loud clicking noise every late afternoon. From her polypharmacy, it was difficult to match symptoms to a particular drug. Her depression was worse than any previous episode in her life. She begged for ECT, and she received treatments 3 times a week for 6 weeks.

A psychiatrist put her on a slew of drugs to manage her symptoms, but the medications all fell short. It was not one day at a time but one hour at a time. She desperately wanted to see William, and unlike most cases, it was thought that William might smooth out her rocky course. At the two-week mark, after the termination, she was stable enough to start her lymphoma treatment.

William planned out his talk with Rona well in advance. Rona looked like she was truly dying. He was far from being shocked. It met his expectations. The only significant problem that he could help Rona with was paying her bills and most of her debt. William lifted her depression to a level that all of her caretakers were surprised to see.

Rona was out for a year. She was sober but never stopped craving the drugs. She was lymphoma-free after that year. She went to meetings three times a week.

One year after discharge, she won teacher of the year in both the department of anesthesia and from the medical school. She was touched and weepy about the awards. Some members of the department who did not know Rona's story took her out to dinner to celebrate. Rona sat at the end of the table and ordered a martini and a second one, and a third one. William gave her a pass and resumed his resolve to keep Rona sober.

By the 18-month mark since Rona detoxed, with the blessing of her psychiatrists, she was ready to go back to work. She contacted Chris, and he agreed to take her on as a Per Diem. She would work Monday–Friday from 6 AM to 3 PM. There were no benefits, and she was not a member of the faculty. She would work alone without the help of residents or CRNAs. Chris would drug test her at a time and as often as he wanted. If she were able to fulfill her responsibilities for a year, a full faculty appointment to the Trinity faculty would be offered.

Rona had three positive drug tests. She appeared to be sober at work, but she was not. Chris had to let her go, but made sure that she could "check back in" at Fairway.

After another year of rehabilitation, Chris helped her secure a position in the pathology residency. Rona embraced this opportunity. Her career in anesthesia was over. The desire to use drugs never went away.

Suggested Reading

1. Anbalagan S, Mendez MD. Neonatal abstinence Syndrome 2023 July 21. In: StatPearls [Internet]. Treasure Island (FL): StatPearls Publishing; 2023 Jan–. PMID: 31855342.
2. Dalmijn EW, Visse MA, van Nistelrooij I. Decision-making in case of an unintended pregnancy: an overview of what is known about this complex process. J Psychosom Obstet Gynaecol. 2024;45(1):2321461. https://doi.org/10.1080/0167482X.2024.2321461. Epub 2024 Mar 12. PMID: 38469857.
3. Grischkan JA, Asch DA. Forgiving physician debt. Ann Intern Med. 2023;176(3):406–7. https://doi.org/10.7326/M22-2832. Epub 2023 Feb 14.PMID: 36780648.

4. Katz JD. The impaired and/or disabled anesthesiologist. Curr Opin Anaesthesiol. 2017;30(2):217–22. https://doi.org/10.1097/ACO.0000000000000423. PMID: 28005618 Review.
5. Young LW, Ounpraseuth ST, Merhar SL, Hu Z, Simon AE, Bremer AA, Lee JY, Das A, Crawford MM, Greenberg RG, Smith PB, Poindexter BB, Higgins RD, Walsh MC, Rice W, Paul DA, Maxwell JR, Telang S, Fung CM, Wright T, Reynolds AM, Hahn DW, Ross J, McAllister JM, Crowley M, Shaikh SK, Puopolo KM, Christ L, Brown J, Riccio J, Wong Ramsey K, Akshatha, Braswell EF, Tucker L, McAlmon KR, Dummula K, Weiner J, White JR, Howell MP, Newman S, Snowden JN, Devlin LA, ACT NOW Collaborative. Eat, sleep, console approach or usual care for neonatal opioid withdrawal. N Engl J Med. 2023;388(25):2326–37. https://doi.org/10.1056/NEJMoa2214470. Epub 2023 Apr 30. PMID: 37125831. Clinical Trial.

To Numb to Push

19

Juliana Wilson

When Juliana Wilson is asked where she is from, the response is always the same "I am from the home of the Apollo Theatre! If I say Harlem, it conjures up thoughts of old school Harlem; horrific crime, rat infestation, drug deals, and an unemployed population. No more!! It is and has been the African-American music and culture in New York City for more than a century!"

The 1964 Freedom Day protest was before Juliana's time. Frustrations with poor education for Black and Puerto Rican students in New York led to a massive protest against segregation. On February 3, 1964, 464,000 New York City school children—almost half of the city's student body—boycotted school as part of a protest against school segregation. This was one of the largest civil rights protests in the history of the entire world.

"I was bused to Stuyvesant and prospered by the policies against segregation. New York remains one of the most segregated cities in the country. A few white parents had strong objections to the admission policies that accepted a number of students by their underserved backgrounds over more qualified white kids. The leadership of our political parties have avoided the issue like the plague. Our diverse country at times is not diverse. There are white people and there is everyone else."

Juliana had younger sisters; all of the siblings considered themselves as middle class. Their parents lived from check to check and were frugal to the extreme. The goal of Juliana's parents was to save enough money to send their kids to college. They fell short of their goal, and the college endeavor would require affirmative action, money, and scholarships.

During Juliana's senior year of high school, her mom was diagnosed with breast cancer with positive axillary nodes. After a mastectomy and immunotherapy, she was, at the moment, disease-free. Her three girls wanted her to stop working as a third-grade teacher in Harlem. Juliana and her two sisters would take care of her.

With the loss of income, they did their homework in the school library and went straight to McDonald's for their shift from 5 to 11. The plan worked out, but exhaustion was there every day. The rigidity of the library made all three better students.

C. Scher, *Anesthesia Conversations*,
https://doi.org/10.1007/978-3-032-05354-1_19

Juliana fit the profile of an Ivy League school candidate, but the tuition, room and board, and daily finances fell well short of the family budget. San Diego State was affordable. It was a perfect fit. Juliana was offered a partial scholarship to keep California's students in California. Room and board were paid for by the state but Juliana had to move into a dorm that was not her choice. She wanted a wheel for ceramics and easels for painting; not a roommate. San Diego State granted her half the rent up to 1000 dollars a month. San Diego State honored Juliana's wish. The school offered her a single room with space for her art projects. Inspired by her mom's doctors, medicine was the only acceptable path for her.

Juliana had been engaged in fine arts since first grade. She could paint, draw, sculpt, weave with a loom, and use her clay and a wheel for ceramic pieces. These skills were passed down and encouraged by her mom. There was a small area in their unfinished basement where Juliana kept the kiln, canvases, a wheel, and canvases that were not yet completed. Their mother also had a sit-down loom to weave. Juliana's fine arts teacher was her mother until the department of fine arts started in middle school. Juliana's creative works were noticed at art shows in LA.

Juliana struggled at San Diego State with a problem that she had never encountered before. She breezed through her classes with a GPA of 3.7. The problem was white people. Her only interaction with white people in her childhood was during her high school years at Stuyvesant. She did not have any white friends there, but did feel respect from students of different cultures and colors. There was no significant social tension in her life in high school.

San Diego State is a public university that has a reputation for having a diverse student body. As a premed student, the competition was fierce. The teachers could not give everyone in the class an A. Tests on premed classes were made to weed out students. Juliana had a reputation for getting A's in most of her classes because she was black. She was devastated by the sentiment. She could not conceive that her academic excellence was being questioned by a significant number of white students. Juliana made an appointment with her student advisor who was black. Her advisor confirmed her sentiment.

"It is what it is. What you are saying is 100% true. Only 5% of the school is either black or African-American. The competition among the white pre-med students brings out the worst in them. Their racist behavior was dormant until you showed up. They think that your 3.77 GPA is based on you being 'privileged'. You will get into several medical schools and they know it. There is nothing that we can do about it. Are you a member of the Black Student Council of BSC African Union? You are now in your fourth year and it is never too late to join. These groups are for solidarity and inclusion. It is highly unlikely, you will feel the tension in medical school. You will make friends in medical school. I am sure of that."

Juliana was accepted to 10 medical schools. Her interest in oncology was very refreshing. She chose NYU. The school was free to all: just show up. After an excellent third-year rotation in anesthesiology, she moved on from oncology. She matched at the Department of Anesthesiology at Duke and chose Tulane for her obstetrical anesthesia fellowship.

Chris was an honorary faculty member at Tulane. He had never "used" his title to better himself. At the beginning of her fellowship, he rounded up his Trinity Obstetrical Anesthesia attendings and fellows for a recruitment dinner at Brigstens to recruit Juliana. Chris asked Juliana to view the department's website.

She looked at the website before she was picked up for dinner.

"Dr. Landry, are there any white people in the residency or faculty?"

"Let me think about that?", the website says it all. We honor DEI.

"Dr Chris, I am all in!"

"Chris, I topped up an epidural with 0.5% Bupivacaine in a patient whose cervix was fully effaced and 8 cm dilated. She is numb and cannot push. The fetal heart tracing is normal, but a C-section is imminent. I gave the 0.5% Bupivacaine 15 minutes ago."

"Julianna, this happens every day in every hospital. Many women of color refuse an epidural for their labor. There are issues with access, trust, culture and the data that people of color have measurable pain despite the epidural. It remains true that they are 'forced by their obstetricians and anesthesiologists' more than white people."

"Today, there is another patient of color; dilated 4 cm and the head at −2 station. She 'lost it' with each contraction."

Juliana offered the patient the epidural, explaining step by step in the process. Although very conflicted, the patient agreed to the epidural.

Juliana automatically called for a midwife. The midwives are highly educated and provide alternative techniques; childbirth education, emotional support, massage, aroma therapy, audio therapy, and the therapeutic use of hot and cold. More advanced techniques include intradermal injections of water, hydrotherapy, transcutaneous electrical injections, acupressure acupuncture, and hypnosis. These techniques cannot be scientifically studied, as each technique has too many confounding variables, but most mothers are pleased with the choice of having a midwife.

Juliana was the backup in this case. She would intervene if there were problematic fetal heart tracings, bleeding, or for any problems that needed a surgical or complex medical intervention. The midwife introduced herself and began applying her craft. The obstetrician rechecked the patient 1 hour after she had first examined the patient. There was no change in station or cervical dilatation. The fetal heart monitor was converted to an internal monitor, and some variable decelerations were on display. The midwife asserted that this was nothing but head compression. The ultrasound was reassuring.

After 2 hours, there was no clear progress. The contractions were organized and extremely painful. The midwife lost control of the patient, and her techniques were not working. Juliana was called to perform a PCA epidural. The concentration of the bupivacaine was 0.5%.was injected. The patient regained her resolve now that she had no pain.

It was time to push. The patient had no pain, no motor function, and a loss of proprioception. Juliana blew it. The dose of 0.5% Bupivacaine was jeopardizing the safety of the birth. The strong local anesthetic was supposed to have worn off, but showed no sign of wearing off. There were three choices: (1) have her push when the fetal heart monitor showed there was a contraction; (2) pull the baby out with forceps; or (3) perform a STAT C-section. Prolonged pushing is associated with sepsis and hemorrhage.

A vaginal delivery with forceps was far hardly desirable yet successful. The obstetrician gave Juliana a mouthful of four-letter words. He told her that he did not want to work with her ever again. Guilt settled in despite an acceptable outcome.

The obstetrician wrote a vitriolic letter to Juliana's Chair, the Designated Institutional Officer, the Chair of Obstetrics and the Dean. He was asking them to have her resign. The pressure on Juliana was brutal.

"An acceptable outcome does not get you off the hook from almost killing the baby." The posting on Facebook by the obstetrician about Juliana was horrific and went viral. He told every one of his colleagues about Juliana's "fuck up." Chris filed a lawsuit against the obstetrician.

"Social media? Really?" Chris asked the obstetrician to resign. The hornet's nest was completely disturbed.

Chris took Juliana off the obstetrical anesthesia service for 4 weeks as per Chris's lawyer. As the dust was settling, Julianna applied for a faculty position at other institutions. Three elite programs offered her interviews. Chris intervened by giving her 3 weeks' paid leave. He did not want Juliana to leave the department.

Two weeks into her leave, she gave notice. She accepted a position at home in New York City. Chris took the blame. He was an ineffective leader when he needed to be effective.

Suggested Reading

1. Głuszak M, FrackGi S, Wielgoś M, Wegrzyn P. Methods of evaluating labor progress in contemporary obstetrics. Ginekol Pol. 2013;84(8):709–13. PMID: 24191505.
2. He F-Y, Wabg S. Epidural analgesia for labor: effects on length of labor and maternal and neonatal outcomes. Eur Rev Med Pharmacol Sci. 2023;27(1):130–7. https://doi.org/10.26355/eurrev_202301_30863. PMID: 36647860.
3. Smith A, Laflamme E, Komanecky C. Pain management and labor. Am Fam Physician. 2021;103(6):355–64. PMID: 33719377.
4. Woznick D, Józefowicz A, Cymbaluk-Płoska A, Kurzawa R. Effect of epidural analgesia on the course of labor. Eur Rev Med Pharmacol Sci. 2023;27(6):2522–34. https://doi.org/10.26355/eurrev_202303_31786. PMID: 370137702.
5. Wright A, Nassar AH, Visser G, Ramasauskaite D, Theron G, FIGO Safe Motherhood and Newborn Health Committee. FIGO good clinical practice paper: management of the second stage of labor. Int J Gynaecol Obstet. 2021;152(2):172–81. https://doi.org/10.1002/ijgo.13552. PMID: 33340411.

Anesthesia for the Eclamptic Parturient 20

Lucas Drachtman

Lucas held a locum tenens position after an obstetrical anesthesiology fellowship at Trinity. He had no interest in an academic position and needed the flexibility afforded by a locum's position. His life outside of medicine was more meaningful inside of medicine. Work simply paid for his wandering mind. He was always at the annual Society for Obstetric Anesthesia and Perinatology Society meeting to see his friends from his residency and fellowship. This year's meeting was in Chicago. He tried to find one of his "amigos" to go to dinner with him at Alinea, a 3 Michelin Star restaurant in Chicago.

Lucas was the ultimate foodie and wanted to meet Chef Grant Achatz, who "paints food" on the table. Lucas guessed you would need a bank loan to dine. He found his buddy, Mike Staley, who was on the Trinity faculty, whom he befriended in their obstetrical anesthesia fellowship. Mike was not married and was the sole beneficiary of his parents' wealth who both passed away 2 years ago. They were buried in Lafayette #1 cemetery, just a block from his house on Second Street.

Over 10 years, Lucas worked with a wealth manager to increase his portfolio with 60% equities to have him retire around 60 years old. that. No woman could possibly derail any part of his predetermined schedule; New Orleans Jazz Fest, Fenway Park, skiing out West, the Paris Open, and concerts at Tanglewood. He savored many of the 3 Michelin Star restaurants in the United States. All flights were first class, and they thought nothing of paying for a hotel for one thousand dollars a night. He did not like to dine alone and always found a woman to join him.

Lucas was not a showoff or a braggart. He dressed like he came out of Paul Stewart and was rarely in jeans. Although he changed into scrubs upon arrival, he always wore a suit on the way out. He was always ready to go to an upscale bar in New Orleans between his next locums. He did not want to marry. He did not want kids. His friends were always "friends for life."

Lucas did not forget a single moment of the fright he felt in their small boat that made the voyage from Havana to Miami. His underwear was packed with jewelry

C. Scher, *Anesthesia Conversations*,
https://doi.org/10.1007/978-3-032-05354-1_20

and cash. There were detailed instructions concerning boat etiquette, which included not making a word on the trip,

There were 10 Cubans on board on a boat that barely fit four. There were four Cuban breads and some cheese. Extreme rationing was the plan. It was expected that the 90-mile trip would feel like 900 miles, and any weather setback could deplete the gasoline that was measured to last 100 miles.

The ocean was the bathroom, and it was two people per blanket. Lucas was 7, and the boat ride would take around 15 hours. He did not sleep for a minute, and everyone on the boat had family or friends waiting for them. Lucas's memory of what happened upon arrival was gone. He was told by his parents that a cousin took his family into his house. By the end of the week after countless Cuban sandwiches (Cuban bread, ham, roasted pork, Swiss cheese, pickles, and mustard), his cousin found an apartment and a job for Lucas's father.

Lucas was an excellent student in the Miami public school system and went on a 100% scholarship to the University of Miami for his undergraduate BS, medical school, and anesthesia residency. His one-year fellowship in obstetrical anesthesia was at Trinity. Lucas jumped around the country as a per diem and a locum. He did not hang around anywhere for more than 3 months. He was a free spirit who wanted to stay free.

Jenna was a 25-year-old G1P0 who presented to her obstetrician for her routine scheduled appointment. Her doctor reviewed her chart, and she was at 30 weeks of gestation. Jena endured the usual obligatory 30-minute wait only to be escorted to a treatment room for another 30 minutes. A physician's assistant entered and took her vitals. Her blood pressure was 173/110. Her pulse was 100, and her voice was notably hoarse. The raspy voice was secondary to edematous vocal cords from the loss of proteins effect on oncotic loss.

A repeat blood pressure was not appreciably different. Bloods were drawn, and a urine sample was submitted. Dr. Hoffman, Jenna's obstetrician, entered the room with a very concerned look on his face. The combination of her hypertension and proteinuria secured the diagnosis of preeclampsia. A systolic pressure greater than 160 and a diastolic pressure greater than or equal to 110 confirmed her diagnosis of severe preeclampsia. Those who are not severe usually do not need hospitalization. Jenna was thrombocytopenic and was tender to abdominal palpation in her right upper quadrant. HELLP was added to the severe preeclampsia diagnosis. HELLP is characterized by hemolysis, elevated liver function tests and low platelets.

Jenna was admitted to the hospital for an infusion of magnesium sulfate to prevent seizures A bolus of 4 grams of magnesium is followed by an infusion of 1–2 grams an hour. The desired magnesium level in severe preeclampsia is 4.8–8.4 mg/dl. Magnesium works concurrently with antihypertensives to release intense vasoconstriction. A balanced salt solution must be administered as the vessels relax.

Historically, hydralazine has been used for blood pressure management for patients with preeclampsia. It is a drug that most anesthesiologists do not use. It is not very titratable. The obstetricians, rightly so, used it as a mainstay, as it has a 100% track record of not harming the fetus. Other classes of antihypertensives are used interchangeably, but ACE inhibitors are absolutely contraindicated. They can be detrimental to the wellness of a fetus; oligohydramnios, fetal renal failure, growth retardation, and possibly fetal death.

The definitive treatment of preeclampsia is to deliver the baby. At 30 weeks' gestation, she needed at least 34 weeks for surfactant to maintain alveolar surface tension. Lungs with surfactant lower incidence of intraventricular hemorrhage, decrease the diagnosis of failure to thrive, and lower the risk of an elevated bilirubin.

There was widespread vasoconstriction in her uterus that led to a series of reactions that were dangerous to Jenna and her baby. Her uterus was now making significantly less prostaglandin, leading to 1. liberation of thromboplastin, 2. fibrin deposition, 3. renal glomerular lesions, and 4. proteinuria. The release of renin from her uterus leads to hypertension and edema.

Current research suggests that preeclampsia may be a pregnancy-induced autoimmune disease. Women with preeclampsia develop antibodies that bind and activate AT1 angiotensin receptors. The antibodies may be similar to those with graft versus host disease. Current research is investigating mRNA and preeclampsia.

The chief resident of ENT was consulted. She used a short nasal fiberoptic scope to evaluate Jenna's hoarse voice. Her vocal cords were moderately to severely edematous from the lack of oncotic protein. This finding was essential when evaluating the safest anesthetic plan.

Lucas examined her lumbar spine, and pitting edema was severe. While it is intuitively obvious that a spinal anesthetic could lead to a rapid onset of hypotension, spinal anesthesia has not been shown to cause more hypotension than an epidural anesthesia in this scenario.

The plan moving forward was a C-section as soon as the baby was 36–37 weeks' gestation, including a resolution of thrombocytopenia. They did not want Jenna to have a trial of labor. The symptoms of preeclampsia resolve after the baby is born or days after the baby is born.

Lucas checked the most recent labs focused on coagulation. The platelet count was 65 thousand. Current guidelines state that the platelet count for an epidural should be 80 thousand and 40 thousand for a spinal.

"I think that we will be fine as is. Cancer patients have spinal taps to inject chemo. Often the counts are 10–20 thousand without neuraxial hematomas.

Let's just go for it. The odds of losing an airway are statistically higher than an epidural hematoma with a platelet count of 65,000."

Jenna sat on the edge of the bed. Her back was prepped and draped with sterile technique. Due to severe edema and adipose tissue, the spinous processes could not be palpated. The resident injected lidocaine at the needle insertion site. Using a loss-of-resistance using saline, the resident made four attempts. He kept hitting bone. Lucas called the anesthesia workroom for a particular ultrasound. Lucas was more proficient with an ultrasound than most. He claimed that he could only find interspaces with the ultrasound.

Lucas sent the resident to the anesthesia workroom for an 8.5-inch epidural needle. Andrew discussed various strategies. The continuous spinal and epidural (CSE) was plan A; a loss of resistance with saline and a 27-gauge spinal needle through the epidural needle to puncture the dura. Hyperbaric bupivacaine (12 mg) along with 25 mcg of fentanyl would be injected through the spinal needle. The spinal needle will be removed, and the epidural catheter would be threaded into the epidural space. This epidural catheter would provide analgesia after the C-section. A "wet" tap during the epidural would take Andrew down an undesirable pathway.

"This is no longer a teaching case." Lucas rarely intervened when a resident was in trouble. He always wanted the resident to "figure it out," but the case was now too complicated and the patient was too sick for resident teaching. Lucas took the epidural needle and "went for it."

Despite the significant lumbar edema, Lucas did see the interspace on ultrasound so that he could proceed. He pushed the needle extremely slowly and had a perfect loss of resistance. He took the syringe off, and a jet of CSF flew onto his scrub shirt. Lucas grabbed the epidural catheter and placed it into the subarachnoid space.

"We now have an anesthetic. I am not disappointed. The epidural catheter will keep CSF from leaking. It will plug the hole and should reduce the chance of a spinal headache."

The big-ticket question was to figure out the spinal dose. The catheter is long. Lucas wanted to test his residency to determine the dose of bupivacaine through a long epidural catheter.

"Do we increase the dose to accommodate the length of the catheter or do we just give the dose we planned through the spinal? It is a rhetorical question. We will administer the original 12 mgs of bupivacaine and 25 mcg of fentanyl super slowly. We can always add if need be."

The next clinical question was "how long do you keep the subarachnoid catheter in, to cause a fibrous reaction around the catheter and prevent a spinal headache." The catheter was pulled on day 3. An awful post-dural puncture headache followed.

On the third postdelivery day, Jenna was found by a group of nursing students, unconscious in her own vomit, and was not responsive. The prevailing thought was that she had a seizure and was now postictal. The other possibility was that Jenna developed cerebral hypotension from the CSF leak. An MRI was ordered to look at both her lumbar spine and head.

There was a large collection of CSF around her spine, and there was no evidence of cerebral hypotension. The brain was buoyant in CSF. Jenna was admitted to the medical intensive care unit. A radial arterial line was inserted. A nicardipine infusion was titrated to a blood pressure no higher than 140 systolic. After 2 days in the intensive care unit, she was admitted to a regular room for two nights before discharge.

Lucas blamed himself for the CSF leak. He also turned the magnesium off at the end of the C-section. He should have given antibiotics for prophylaxis for the intrathecal catheter, but he did not.

He did not take a few minutes out of his day to round on the patient at the end of the day. By dividing his time, where a life outside of the hospital far exceeded his life in the hospital was the reason that Lucas was no longer current in his practice. He did not feel shame, embarrassment, or guilt. It was a teaching case for the resident who will never forget Lucas's disconnect from the patient "way to early."

Suggested Reading

1. Altman D, Carroli G, Duley L, Farrell B, Moodley J, Neilson J, Smith D, Magpie Trial Collaboration Group. Do women with pre-eclampsia, and their babies, benefit from magnesium sulphate? The Magpie Trial: a randomised placebo-controlled trial. Lancet. 2002;359(9321):1877–90. https://doi.org/10.1016/s0140-6736(02)08778-0. PMID: 12057549.
2. Hauspurg A, Jeyabalan A. Postpartum preeclampsia or eclampsia: defining its place and management among the hypertensive disorders of pregnancy. Am J Obstet Gynecol. 2022;226(2S):S1211–21. https://doi.org/10.1016/j.ajog.2020.10.027. Epub 2021 Jul 7. PMID: 35177218.
3. Ives CW, Sinkey R, Rajapreyar I, Tita ATN, Oparil S. Preeclampsia-pathophysiology and clinical presentations: JACC state-of-the-art review. J Am Coll Cardiol. 2020;76(14):1690–702. https://doi.org/10.1016/j.jacc.2020.08.014. PMID: 33004135.
4. Moore JM. Continuous spinal anesthesia. Am J Ther. 2009;16(4):289–94. https://doi.org/10.1097/MJT.0b013e3181729d2a. PMID: 19546804 Review.
5. Palei AC, Spradley FT, Warrington JP, George EM, Granger JP. Pathophysiology of hypertension in pre-eclampsia: a lesson in integrative physiology. Acta Physiol (Oxf). 2013;208(3):224–33. https://doi.org/10.1111/apha.12106. Epub 2013 May 7. PMID: 23590594.
6. Palmer CM. Continuous spinal anesthesia and analgesia in obstetrics. Anesth Analg. 2010;111(6):1476–9. https://doi.org/10.1213/ANE.0b013e3181f7e3f4. Epub 2010 Oct 1.

21 Epidural Anesthesia Complicated by Subarachnoid Cutaneous Fistula

Tim Norris

Tim Norris was the class nerd and became the most popular and unique resident in his class. He started his Ochsner anesthesia residency when he was 25 and looked like a 55-year-old. At 5 feet 11 inches, he was just shy of 140 pounds. With thinning hair, lack of hair on his entire body, and a face riddled with anxiety, his voice was just above a whisper. His sunglasses were always on, and his skin was as white as white can be.

With Tim's self-deprecating humor and a brain that held thousands of jokes, his co-residents could look past his gaunt and sickly body. He did not drink nor participate with friends who used weed. Tim's nails were yellow, and he still smoked cigarettes. He never tried to stop. It kept him even.

While no one in the class believed him. He had been a backup quarterback at the University of Iowa. There was a picture of him, in his wallet, pacing the sidelines of a game against Mizzou. The face barely resembled the Tim that his residents knew. He bragged about the archive of photos of him quarterbacking in a game against Iowa State. Impossible.

Tim "fell apart" during his internship, which took him 2 years to complete. He claimed that there was a tragedy in his life that made a full-time, one-year commitment to a surgical internship: impossible to complete. He had months of wellness that were replaced by months of not being well.

The University of Iowa School of Medicine gave him 100% support to work when he could and be on leave as much as he needed. They were more than aware of his decline that started in medical school. Tim loved his life until his life no longer loved him. He never would "fess up" to anyone that he had Crohn's disease.

Tim wanted a job at Trinity. Chris was shocked. He did not know Tim personally, but Tim had become the center of attention in the department rumor mill. Several Trinity faculty members heard of him. They knew that he had been dating Laura in a long-distance relationship for years.

He had a cane to support his right hip. Baldness, cachexia, and his wire-frame glasses made him look like his days were numbered. Chris arranged an itinerary to

C. Scher, *Anesthesia Conversations*,
https://doi.org/10.1007/978-3-032-05354-1_21

meet with all of the chiefs of the divisions of the surgical department. The unlit cigarette spread and general appearance raised the bar of sympathy as he went to each meeting.

Tim could read the room, and it was time to inject some humor with each encounter. His handshake was accompanied by a pat on the back which was not expected. He whispered something in the ears of each Chief that made them hysterical.

Tim opened up his backpack and pulled out a Nike football. He walked into the hall outside the office of the Chief of Orthopedics. The Chief walked around 20 yards down the hall. Tim threw a rocket-like pass, which landed in the gut of the Chief. Tim lost his balance from the throw but was able to grab his cane that was parked by his feet. There was no doubt that this "dying" man had played football at a very high level.

After his Ochsner residency, Tim entered the obstetrical anesthesia fellowship at the University of Alabama in Birmingham. Tim was a planner and wanted to secure a faculty position back home in New Orleans. He firmly believed that his health would be restored after Drago's grilled oysters, Acme Gumbo, a pecan waffle at the Camellia Grill, and a pair of blue soft-shell crabs from Clancy's. After 6 months at Trinity, he was in remission.

A 22-year-old G1PO was in labor. Her cervix was 4 cm, and the baby's head was at the −1 station. She was examined by her obstetrician and was told that it was a perfect time to get an epidural. Her past medical history was entirely normal. She had no surgeries and never had an anesthetic. Her BMI was 23, and the landmarks for an epidural could not have been better. Pitocin augmented the pain of each contraction, and the fetal heart tracing was normal. Tim's resident, Tracy, was a senior resident with the most obstetrical anesthesia training in the residency.

The patient was placed in the sitting position, and the epidural space was entered with a loss of resistance with saline. A rush of fluid came out of the Tuohy syringe, and it was clear that the resident had punctured the dura. The needle was removed, and the epidural space was found the second time without incident. The catheter was passed, and a test dose was negative.

A post-dural puncture headache manifested itself as a positional neck ache. The second epidural worked well, but the neck pain was more than bothersome. The explanation of the neck pain comforted the patient, and further treatment of her neck ache would be addressed after the baby was born.

The anesthesia care team responded when the patient's neck pain evolved to a severe post-dural puncture headache. The back of the patient was examined. The epidural catheter was removed with the tip intact. The "wet tap" puncture site was leaking CSF at the skin at a rate that Tim had not seen before. An abdominal binder, and the placement of an ostomy bag over the leaking puncture site was measured every half hour. The conservative therapy was reevaluated the next morning. The ostomy bag had 75 cc of an ongoing leak. The normal amount of CSF in the subarachnoid space is 125–150 cc. The 75 cc in the band was more than significant. The diagnosis of a subdural/subarachnoid cutaneous fistula was made. Tim did a literature review looking at treatment plans. There was a paucity in the literature of cases, and there was no consensus for treatment. The plan was now a blood patch and a skin suture. Vancomycin and Cefepime were ordered to prevent meningitis.

Twenty-four hours later, the patient consented for an epidural blood patch to be placed after the morning conference. During the conference, the overhead speaker announced a "code blue" on the obstetrical floor. Tim and two residents flew down three flights of stairs. They knew it was the patient with the "wet tap."

She was having a full-blown seizure, choking on the stomach contents that were pouring out of her mouth. The ostomy bag over the site of the tap had increased by 100 cc since resident's morning rounds. Tim, always cool and calm, was convinced that this was cerebral hypotension with the diencephalon heading toward the foramen magnum. Tim administered 200 mg of propofol to stop the seizure and a double dose of rocuronium to facilitate an endotracheal intubation.

The residents positioned the patient to the left lateral by flexing the neck and pulling her legs toward her chest. The resident started an epidural while Tim was prepping the arm for a blood draw. When the resident found the epidural space with a loss of resistance to air, Tim handed the resident a 20 cc syringe of blood. The full syringe of blood was injected through the needle without incident. Tim then put 2 nylon stitches through the skin to keep more CSF from dripping out and turned the patient supine. A 500-mg dose of Sugammadex allowed the neurologists to perform a thorough exam after extubation. Thirty minutes after extubation, the patient was 100% neurologically intact, and it appeared that nothing had happened. Tim and his resident stopped a brain herniation. In their debrief, they said that doing an epidural blood patch immediately after delivery might have been helpful in preventing cerebral hypotension and a diencephalic storm. A diencephalic storm is characterized by episodic, intense surges of the sympathetic nervous system. The true storm was prevented by the blood patch and skin sutures. A CT scan revealed a paucity of CSF and a loss of buoyancy of the brain. An EVD was placed to monitor cerebral hypotension.

Chris heard about the football pass and thought it was a tale that was overstated. He could not afford taking an attending on board who was chronically ill. In his experience, the chronically ill were not to be depended on. Chris invited Tim for a drink and pleaded with him to bring his football. Chris wanted to assess his physical strength and endurance.

"Of course we want you on our faculty. No ifs ands or buts. It will take about 1 month to credential you. When you start, you will be accompanied by Billy Murray. He is one of our best all-around faculty members. He will serve as your 'resident' so you learn our system well without stress. Every faculty member gets the same salary, one which you will feel comfortable with. The call system is completely optional. The call person does a 7PM to 7AM call; a night float so to speak. After that week, you get one week off. We do not incentivize with money because, as you clearly see, we do not have much so we give time. The difference is in the benefits that faculty participate in. They are better than most institutions. The salary is 500,000 dollars a year. If you choose to take a week of night float, the only thing the School of Medicine demands is that you cannot give anesthesia somewhere else."

"I most certainly want the job. I will sign the contract as soon as I get it. No need the advice or any other comments from the outside world."

"It will be ready tomorrow. Let's have lunch together. I will meet you at the Palace Cafe on Canal. Of course if you have a significant other, then that will make three of us."

"There is a significant other but she is tied up for tomorrow. I'm looking forward to it. Thank you Chris!"

Suggested Reading

1. Lobo G, Lobo SRJ. Postoperative CSF leak: blood patch-a new avenue. Asian J Neurosurg. 2023;18(4):761–3. https://doi.org/10.1055/s-0043-1768599. eCollection 2023 Dec. PMID: 38161614.
2. Louraoui SM, Fliyou F, Aasfara J, El Azhari A. Paroxysmal sympathetic hyperactivity after traumatic brain injury: what is important to know? Cureus. 2022;14(5):e24693. https://doi.org/10.7759/cureus.24693. eCollection 2022 May. PMID: 35663695.
3. Sanha M, Vaz I, Barbosa H, Alves S, Paiva M. Cerebrospinal fluid cutaneous fistula following neuraxial anesthesia for cesarean delivery. Cureus. 2022;14(12):e32895. https://doi.org/10.7759/cureus.32895. eCollection 2022 Dec. PMID: 36699750.
4. Uppal V, Russell R, Sondekoppam RV, Ansari J, Baber Z, Chen Y, DelPizzo K, Dirzu DS, Kalagara H, Kissoon NR, Kranz PG, Leffert L, Lim G, Lobo C, Lucas DN, Moka E, Rodriguez SE, Sehmbi H, Vallejo MC, Volk T, Narouze S. Evidence-based clinical practice guidelines on postdural puncture headache: a consensus report from a multisociety international working group. Reg Anesth Pain Med. 2024;49(7):471–501. https://doi.org/10.1136/rapm-2023-104817. PMID: 37582578.

22 The Total Spinal

Leonardo "Leo" Vincenza

In 2007, having a baby before a couple gets married was no longer uncommon. Cynthia Ross traveled with her fiancé, Leonardo, to Paris for a romantic vacation. Leonardo popped the question across from the iconic Notre Dame, and within 3 months, Cynthia was pregnant.

When the baby arrived, all hell broke loose in their private lives. Breastfeeding, changing diapers, and bouts of crying for reasons that were not apparent exhausted Cynthia. A touch of postpartum blues augmented the whole event.

Cynthia was in the same medical school class as Leonardo. They started dating while both were in medical school, and both were together on their third-year elective in anesthesia. They did a couple's match and landed at the University of Alabama-Birmingham Department of Anesthesia. Leo went to a neurosurgery anesthesia fellowship at Trinity while Cynthia enrolled at Tulane for a Master's in Clinical Research.

Leo was born at Touro Hospital in New Orleans. His grandfather Saul and father, Archibald, owned two antique stores on the iconic Royal Street in the Vieux Carre, or as the tourists say, the "French Quarter." His father was on the Sewage and Water Board and refused to run for mayor as suggested by the outgoing mayor.

Leo's parents bought a revival Victorian home on Coliseum Street with six bedrooms to accommodate Leo and his three sisters. His father dry-walled off the third floor as an apartment for Leo, Cynthia, and their baby. His two sisters lived in a shotgun on Danneel Street which was the family's second home. They owned a third home on Napoleon Avenue on the Mississippi River side of the city. It was for sale and was on the market for 6 months, until his father took the for sale sign away.

Leo wanted to work at Trinity. He called Chris, and Chris's secretary arranged a lunch for Leo and Cynthia at Joey K's. It was a jeans-and-tee-shirt joint with a roux that was heavy on the okra. Leo scored some points for Chris for picking Joey K's. Leo's uncle opened the restaurant in 1989. The restaurant's classic offerings include red beans and rice, white beans and pork chop, beef brisket, and chicken cordon bleu. It was Friday, and Chris was fired up for the all-you-can-eat Catfish. Leo and

C. Scher, *Anesthesia Conversations*,
https://doi.org/10.1007/978-3-032-05354-1_22

Cynthia were a perfect fit for Trinity. They became Chris's closest confidants over the years.

Leo worked fast and efficiently. He was known in the department for his seamless skills. He never had a "wet tap" or a failed nerve block. Leo was often called to do a procedure when an attending was unsuccessful or struggling. He was the department's fixer.

Cynthia went into labor after 38 weeks of gestation. Her labor was complicated by several episodes of late decelerations. Her physical exam revealed a 4-cm dilated cervix, with the baby's head above the ischial spines at −2 station. Her diagnosis at that time was failure to progress with episodes with non-reassuring fetal heart rates. The obstetricians and pediatricians agreed on a C-section.

Leo insisted that he be the anesthesiologist. Rather than have a scene, Lucas texted Chris who came bolting down to the labor and delivery floor. Chris uttered a comment to Leo which shut him up and Leo came to his senses: "not happening! We never take care of our family members!

Lucas, text me when they are closing."

Leo behaved like a new father, dropping the role of being an overbearing anesthesiologist. Cynthia was petite at 64 inches and 110 pounds, and it took less than 5 minutes to do the spinal. In the sitting position, 12 mg of hyperbaric bupivacaine and 15 micrograms of fentanyl at the L3L4 interspace were injected. It was a one-stick spinal. After 2 minutes, Cynthia was placed in the supine position with a bag of saline under the right hip to keep the baby off the vena cava. Leo was allowed to enter the operating, after the spinal was completed.

The level of the anesthetic was at T4; perfect! Within 2 minutes after the incision, Cynthia complained of a "stuffy" nose and difficulty breathing. She was encouraged to concentrate on breathing with the explanation that she had lost proprioception of her chest wall, and all was well. After 30 seconds, she started to whisper and then lost consciousness.

Lucas grabbed a laryngoscope and an endotracheal tube for intubation. Cynthia's blood pressure was 60/42. The light on the laryngoscope would not turn on. A second scope was not stocked. Lucas grabbed a number 4 I-Gel LMA, and with great force, he seated the I-Gel. The obstetrical team fired questions concerning Cynthia's status. Cynthia had a total spinal.

Cynthia had a safe airway, but Leonardo was overwhelmed, "just get my fucking baby out!"

Four minutes into the section, the baby was born. The anesthesia team was pouring in Lactated Ringers, along with a total of 50 mg of ephedrine and 300 mcg of phenylephrine intravenously. Leo put the table in severe reverse Trendelenburg to allow bupivacaine to leave the brain. This made Cynthia more hypotensive with blood pooling in her legs and brain. Lucas leveled out the bed. The usual uterotonics were administered, and norepinephrine was loaded on a pump and activated at 10 mcg per minute.

Several working laryngoscopes were brought to intubate. Lucas was insisting to intubate and remove the LMA to get a "more stable airway."

Leo was now exasperated. "She is on volume control ventilation and there is no air leak. We have an airway, leave it alone." There are countless reports in the literature on LMAs used for C-sections

As crazy as it sounds, "How long does it take for the total spine to recede so that you can remove the LMA?"

Lucas had seen three total spinals in his fellowship. Typically, the total spinal condition lasts two to four hours. Spontaneous breathing could come back within two hours. Sevoflurane was replaced with a propofol/remi infusion. Sugammadex was administered for rocuronium reversal.

Lucas and Leon agreed to employ the normal criteria for LMA removal. "Just leave everything as is. Leave her be. Again, leave the fucking LMA alone." Leo was now in charge.

Chris came down from his office and was briefed by Lucas. "What the F happened?" Lucus gave his analysis.

"There are several possibilities: Was the dosing miscalculated? Was the speed of the injection too fast? They could have Cynthia lie down right after the injection? The bed was in mild Trendelenburg and finally," I do not know.

After 90 minutes, Cynthia met all of the criteria for LMA removal. Four milligrams of ondansetron 4 mg and 0.6 mg of hydromorphone were administered. Her pulse oximeter read 100%, and the LMA was removed. Other than a pain score of six, Cynthia was safe and well.

Suggested Reading

1. de Sá Oliveira RR, Módolo MP, Mizubuti GB, Ho AMH, de Barros GAM, Muniz da Silva L, Braz LG, Módolo NSP, Day AG, Phelan R, Navarro E, Lima LH, Ganem EM. Total spinal anesthesia failure: have you assessed the sensory anesthesia in sacral dermatomes? Anesth Analg. 2017;124(5):1674–7. https://doi.org/10.1213/ANE.00000000000019. PMID: 28431.
2. Han B, Xu M. Effect of continuous spinal anesthesia on the hemodynamics of labor analgesia in hypertensive pregnant women: a comparative, randomized trial. BMC Anesthesiol. 2023;23(1):205. https://doi.org/10.1186/s12871-023-02174-1. PMID: 37312032 Clinical Trial.
3. Hussein K, Patel H, Drew T. Total spinal anaesthesia and respiratory arrest during patient transfer following unrecognised subdural catheter placement during labour. Int J Obstet Anesth. 2023;53:103621. https://doi.org/10.1016/j.ijoa.2022.103621. Epub 2022 Dec 23. PMID: 36634447.
4. Kumar CM, Seet EE. Continuous spinal technique in surgery and obstetrics. Best Pract Res Clin Anaesthesiol. 2023;37(2):139–56. https://doi.org/10.1016/j.bpa.2023.02.007. Epub 2023 Mar. PMID: 37321763.
5. She YJ, Liu WX, Wang LY, Ou XX, Liang HH, Lei DX. The impact of height on the spread of spinal anesthesia and stress response in patients undergoing cesarean section: a prospective observational study. BMC Anesthesiol. 2021;21(1):298. https://doi.org/10.1186/s12871-021-01523. PMID: 34847868.

"Death by the Epidural"

23

Rick Fromer, Peter Lichtenstein

The obstetrical floor was very busy with six women in labor. Peter Lichtenstein had two residents, and all of the patients had reassuring fetal heart tracings. Two of the patients had two preexisting epidurals from the shift before. There were two more that had to be placed.

Peter Lichtenstein had a pedigree education. His more than impressive CV listed an undergraduate degree from Dartmouth, medical school at Albert Einstein, and an anesthesia residency at the University of Pittsburgh. He chose not to do a fellowship and was self-taught in regional anesthesia.

The main operating room was quiet, and Peter texted Chris to send another resident to help out. Rick Fromer had already accepted a fellowship in cardiac anesthesia at Phoenix Heart. He performed anesthesia at the level of an experienced attending. Peter was relieved that Rick was sent to him for help during a very busy time of day.

Fathers were allowed to stay in the patient's room for epidural placement. Rick explained to the laboring mother and father. The process of placing an epidural. All the father had to do was stand in front of his sitting wife and keep her from moving when she was having a contraction. What was puzzling to Peter and his residents was that there were two doors in a patient's room. There was a door to walk into the patient's room and a door across the room to get out.

In most cases, the epidural was placed, and medications were part of a PCEA pump set up with various algorithms. When the patient was in pain, the patient had to press a button, and a pump would inject medication into the epidural catheter. Rick had excellent hands and placed the epidural in ten minutes, and all was well.

Rick then proceeded to the next epidural. The father, a bundle of nerves, did not want to be in the room for the epidural placement. His fears got the best of him, and he and the rest of the family paced outside the room nervously, wondering what was taking so long to put an epidural in?

They waited 20 minutes and then barged in without knocking. Dr. Fromer was gone, and the patient was blue, and taking slow, shallow breaths. The EKG

C. Scher, *Anesthesia Conversations*,
https://doi.org/10.1007/978-3-032-05354-1_23

displayed a heart rate of ten. The father started CPR, and the family screamed out for help. With the baby on the vena cava, it is extremely difficult to be successful following the ACLS algorithms.

Peter, who was with the family, entered the room and screamed "anesthesia STAT in room 224." Rick stormed into the room, and Peter was well into CPR. Peter intubated the patient, and the nurses did chest compressions. Rick administered two rounds of epinephrine. The patient alternated between asystole and ventricular fibrillation. With no progress with CPR, Peter called for a stat section to save the baby. By the time they entered the OR, the patient had pulseless electrical activity, and CPR continued for the entire C-section.

The baby was delivered 4 minutes after the skin incision. The APGAR score of the baby was 2/4. The baby was transferred to the neonatal ICU for intensive care by the neonatologists. The mother required multiple doses of emergency drugs and was declared dead 45 minutes from when she was found "down" after the epidural.

When an epidural is placed, it is tested to determine if the tip of the catheter is in the subarachnoid space or in a blood vessel. Two drugs (test dose) are administered from a single vial into the new epidural. If the catheter is in a vessel, the epinephrine in the test solution would raise the heart rate by at least 10 beats per minute. If the tip of the catheter was in the spinal fluid, the patient would have a low spinal (Numbness no higher than the umbilicus)

After the RCA, Rick did not do a test dose. Rick did not stay in the room long enough to evaluate the safety of the epidural. Rick went out the second door, the back door, as it was called in the RCA. He did not talk to the family after he completed the epidural. The conclusion from the RCA committee was that Rick administered the entire epidural dose of bupivacaine into a blood vessel. Bupivacaine is a sodium channel blocker that stops the heart. Intralipid was never ordered.

The case went to court. Rick and Peter pleaded not guilty, as there was no evidence, only speculation that the epidural was the cause of death. It is common practice that senior residents can work alone in their final year.

The jury's conclusive verdict came after all of the facts were presented and dissected. Rick was guilty of a second degree manslaughter, reckless abandonment, lack of knowledge of the efficacy of intralipid, and unprofessional behavior at the highest level. A healthy 20-year-old should never die during a normal labor. This was the ultimate breach of anesthetic care.

The judge moved quickly on the sentence. Rick was sentenced for one year in prison, fined two million dollars, and permanently suspended from his medical license with no parole. Peter received the same sentence.

Suggested Reading

1. Caplan RA, Ward RJ, Posner K, Cheney FW. Unexpected cardiac arrest during spinal anesthesia: a closed claims analysis of predisposing factors. Anesthesiology. 1988;68(1):5–11. https://doi.org/10.1097/00000542-198801000-00003. PMID: 3337390.

2. Jung S, McDowell RH. Abandonment. In: StatPearls [Internet]. Treasure Island (FL): StatPearls Publishing; 2022. 2023 Jan–. PMID: 33085432.
3. Lee SH, Sohn JT. Mechanisms underlying lipid emulsion resuscitation for drug toxicity: a narrative review. Korean J Anesthesiol. 2023;76(3):171–82. https://doi.org/10.4097/kja.23031. Epub 2023 Jan 26. PMID: 36704816.
4. Massoth C, Wenk M. Epidural test dose in obstetric patients. Should we still use it? Curr Opin Anaesthesiol. 2019;32(3):263–7.
5. Souter KJ, Gallagher TH. The disclosure of unanticipated outcomes of care and medical errors: what does this mean for anesthesiologists. Anesth Analg. 2012;114(3):615–21. https://doi.org/10.1213/ANE.0b013e3182228604. Epub 2011 Jun 3. PMID: 21642607 Review.
6. Van Norman GA. A matter of life and death: what every anesthesiologist should know about the medical, legal, and ethical aspects of declaring brain death. Anesthesiology. 1999;91(1):275–87. https://doi.org/10.1097/00000542-199907000-00036. PMID: 10422953.

24 Not All Anesthesiologists Who Become Addicted Are the Same

William Robinson

William Robinson was the faculty "Golden Boy": an undergraduate at Notre Dame, medical school at Cornell, an anesthesia residency at the University of North Carolina, and a neuroanesthesia fellowship at LSU New Orleans. Chris knew William well and recruited him to be the head of the Neuroanesthesia division.

As a medical student and Chief Resident at UNC, he published two sentinel papers. Both generated research that generated 20 peer-reviewed papers. William was married and had two children and was divorced after 4 years of marriage. He could not clean up his mess.

The 24-hour call during residency was brutal at UNC. An hour or two of sleep or more likely none, while on call, did nothing for his dysphoria, depressed mood, and exhaustion that started the minute he arrived home from a bone-crushing all-nighter. Most residents were showered and asleep within the first hour of arriving home. William was afflicted with the inability to sleep after being on his feet for over 24 hours. He wasted his time going to the sleep clinic. His greatest fear was not being able to sleep and was now facing another call the next day. That fear of not sleeping remained with him for the rest of his life.

He was not unnoticed by his colleagues. His physical appearance changed dramatically. His sculpted body became gaunt, with uncombed hair and a full ratty beard. His teeth were now yellow from his new hobby: non-filtered cigarettes. His wife begged him to take a leave and get help. Despite the look of a man who was truly suffering, there was no doubt that he was "one of the best residents with sincerity and compassion for his patients."

How much more could he take before he collapsed? William arranged a meeting with the Chief Resident of Psychiatry. The psychiatry resident listened to William's story, which he had heard countless times from other residents in other career paths: exhaustion, despair, and depression, all from a lack of sleep.

The psych residents had a uniform prescription book, which was registered with the Drug Enforcement Agency. The scripts had a piece of carbon paper underneath to keep records of each script. Electronic prescriptions had not arrived in North

C. Scher, *Anesthesia Conversations*,
https://doi.org/10.1007/978-3-032-05354-1_24

Carolina and Louisiana. There were countless ways of diverting drugs with this precomputer statewide system that existed in most states.

Most psych residents had their own prescription pads that were perfectly designed with the aid of a printer. The psych resident pulled out of his backpack his private pad. "Jack Rothstein MD." Jack wrote William a prescription for Diazepam, 5 mg #60. Jack instructed William to start at 5 mg and wait 45 minutes, and if that did not work, take another 5 mg.

The pills worked like magic; ten uninterrupted hours of sleep followed by a sumptuous breakfast. He ran to the bathroom for a shower and a shave. He was alive again! His normally good mood was restored and took his pills when he came home for a call. He slept for 6 hours on the post-call day and turned on his DVD player and binged-watched movies. After a month, he would sleep till noon and hit the basketball courts. In the late afternoon, William made himself a generous martini without spilling a drop. He ordered Chinese food and reasoned that if he ate early, his stomach would be empty for the 2 pills of diazepam. William called Jack to thank him for literally saving his life.

William was not a patient, yet Jack wrote scripts for 6 months. Jack was guilty of not keeping medical records while prescribing a benzodiazepine. His carbon copy of his scripts was questioned by the psychiatry program director. It was time to inform William that he needed to move on. To dissect Jack's activities, he was unknowingly created an addict. Jack said that it is better to be on sleeping pills than be totally exhausted without restorative sleep.

Jack was preaching a philosophy that many psychiatrists believed. The mantra among some "shrinks" was once on a benzo, you bought it for life. The process of detoxification and restoration of well-being was so tumultuous and long that it was a cost–benefit decision to quit versus a low dose forever. There was no research at that time about how chronic benzo use can lead to neurodegeneration in the brain.

Diazepam is not a sleeping pill. It is used for many ailments, but tolerance is the rule. The amount that William would need to sleep increased fivefold. William became a pill counter. When there were ten left in the vial it was time to go into action. Jack was aware that weaning should be slow and supervised.

William found a print shop in the Central Business Department with ease. Within minutes, his problem was solved. A prescription pad with a made-up name, address, and phone number was ready for prime time. He put a fake medical license number on it and a line to sign on. There was a shield at the top of the script that conveyed power. William made up his first script.

The patient's name was Charles Baptiste. The script was: diazepam 5 mg #60 Sig: 1–2 tabs qhs (hour of sleep). He dropped it off at a mom-and-pop pharmacy and told the pharmacist in Abita that he would pay in cash. He would never go to the same pharmacy more than once.

William planned to spend weekends making big scores with his pad. He rented a car on a Friday after work. With his map of rural South Carolina, he hit 10 small pharmacies just 20 miles from Charleston. By 5 PM on Saturday, he had 300 pills.

The exact same problem was solved in New Orleans. During his time in New Orleans, he hit the local New Orleans pharmacies and scored another 300 pills.

Each script was priced at around 20 dollars. The following weekend included President's Day. He collected pills from Marrero, Metairie, Abita, Covington, and Kenner. The pill count was now 1200. This was still not enough in William's mind.

William was exhausted from fear and lying. His last score was from four rural towns near Jackson, Mississippi. His grand total was 1500: enough for the year.

William's wife knew what he was doing but thought that this was not a better William. She insisted that he see a psychiatrist. She was aware that the pill "scam" was illegal. She suggested supervised weaning. William shot that down her proposal ASAP. He would live his life with diazepam. His wife's suggestions simply made William livid. "You just do not understand!? He did not have the insight to see that his addiction and marriage were not sustainable. He was a junkie, and he could not see further than a 5 mg tablet of diazepam.

After 2 years of this maladaptive behavior, the phone call finally arrived. The man on the phone introduced himself as an investigator for the Drug Enforcement Agency, and William rapidly lost his shit. He slammed the phone down on the kitchen counter.

"Oh my god, they are going to take my license away. They will surely throw me out of the department!! My activity is criminal and I could end up in a prison."

William did not know, but the officer on the phone was from the DEA and was simply calling to report to providers the dangers of prescribing codeine. Codeine is broken down into morphine, which could be a serious problem for children if prescribed for a cough. William was in such a state that he did not process the information from the officer. There was no mention of William's drug diversion.

His wife left William and took their kids to live with his wife's mother. She could not take William's maladaptive behavior anymore and filed for divorce. There was no one in her family that thought Williams's behavior would end well. She thought William would never recover. She spoke to social workers, psychologists, psychiatrists, and addiction counselors. His addiction put him first and his family last.

The divorce went through very quickly. Her claims were that William was not fit to be a father or husband. William knew that his wife was correct on every account and acquiesced. William had lost everything: his wife, children, and some friends in the know. In a moment of self-loathing, he gathered up all of the diazepam in the house, hundreds of pills, and flushed them down the toilet. He knew that tough times were coming and called in sick.

William was unable to fall asleep on the third night. Panic was now relentless. By day four, he was manic. There was an open bottle of Ketel One, and he decided to just chug it down. He popped a movie into his DVR and settled in, waiting for the vodka to kick. He felt no change after an hour. Wiliam was now frantic, anxious, manic, and in danger.

William was now at hour 96. Audio hallucinations, dry heaves, and a migraine-like headache found a home in his brain. He was so self-absorbed, and he was not aware that he had not peed in 3 days. Acute kidney disease from profound dehydration was settling in. He remembered that he had a secret place in the living room with a vial of 30 pills. He needed a few pills to end his symptoms and get help. He could not concentrate and find the pills. He checked the vase over the fireplace. They were not there. He had lost his focus.

William had a close friend who lived in an apartment across the street. She was the patient treated by William at Trinity. He was her anesthesiologist for her appendectomy.

Anne was a talented government public defender who was trying a case in Jefferson Parish. William met Anne after she woke up from her anesthesia. They met in the PACU, and William asked her out. He could not put the pieces together when she told him she was a government lawyer who worked on drug-related crimes.

Anne had not seen William in 6 days and was concerned. Of late, when William was not at the gym or in the hospital, they were with each other. He did not respond to her phone calls. She sensed that something was horrifically wrong and went to his apartment and rang the bell, hoping he would answer the door.

Anne had a set of William's keys and opened his door. William had a large one-bedroom condo with an eat-in kitchen. He was supine, breathing and unresponsive. She found a radial artery pulse and called 911.

First responders have a protocol for choosing hospitals depending on the condition of the patient. To protect his privacy, the responders, and to Anne's dismay, they took William to Trinity Hospital; Anne called for help from her car that was in front of the doors to the emergency room.

An intravenous was started, and a liter of Lactated Ringers flowed in. Oxygen was delivered by face mask. A nasogastric tube was passed to aspirate any contents. He remained on the spine board with his neck supported with a cervical spine collar. He was given an intramuscular injection of naloxone. There was no response. A Foley catheter was passed through his penis to collect urine for a toxicology screen, analysis, and urinary output. After a liter of fluid, there was no fluid in the collection bag attached to the catheter.

Ten tubes of blood were sent to the lab for multiple investigatory panels. CT scan of the head demonstrated a right parietal lobe nondepressed linear skull fracture. There was a small pocket of subarachnoid blood adjacent to the skull fracture, and otherwise, there were no other positive signs on the scan. His pupils were equally reactive to light and were of normal size. The patella tendon was hyperreflexed.

Anne was fully informed by William concerning his diazepam addiction soon after his divorce. The information did not make her run. He promised he would take ownership of his problem and stop. Anne filled in the doctors and nurses on his addiction. The ER nurse suggested that either William overdosed or he had a seizure, as commonly described in those who abruptly stopped a benzo. Both hypotheses fit the CT scan reading by a radiologist for the skull fracture.

A dose of flumazenil was brought up by the head of emergency services to reverse the effects of diazepam if he overdosed. There was concern among every provider in the emergency room who was there to help William. Anne put her foot down, and with no medical training, she was stressed out by the proposed plan. She knew that flumazenil was outright bold and dangerous. Flumazenil, the reversal of a benzo, would abruptly bring out the dangers of a rapid detox. William could seize, possibly aspirate, and become psychotic. The order for flumazenil was canceled.

Anne suggested an admission, an addiction psychiatrist for a full evaluation, and a very slow wean from the diazepam. That became the plan.

The anesthesia team was called to intubate William since he was obtunded and no longer could protect his airway. The emergency room physicians did not want William intubated. They were exasperated with the anesthesia team's recommendation, but anesthesia insisted on the intubation. His vital signs hovered around B/P 140 s/90 and a pulse of 110. His temperature was 36.4 and he was breathing at 25/ breaths/minute. 100 mg of Esmolol was administered to prevent an elevation of intracranial pressure from the intubation. A rapid sequence induction of lidocaine, 150 mg of propofol, and 120 mg of rocuronium (double dose) facilitated an easy intubation. A bed was ready for him in the medical intensive care unit. Infusions of dexmedetomidine and remifentanil kept William's vital signs stable. The plan was to keep him asleep for 4 hours and repeat the CT scan. The scan would determine if William had intracranial hypertension from the already pre-existing bleed.

There was no change in the scan, and the anesthetic infusions were discontinued. Blood work was significant for a potassium of 2.8, presumably from vomiting. After the second scan, William woke up, bucking on his endotracheal tube, and was clearly awake. After oral suctioning, William was extubated and was seemingly just ok. The final diagnosis was a seizure from the rapid discontinuance of diazepam.

William had one of two paths that would determine his future. Since what he had done was illegal. He would have to deal with the law or he could just go to rehab. He chose rehab. The process was explained, and William knew that he needed a leave of absence. Anne suggested his absence was due to Lyme's disease. They would sit well with his colleagues and Chris.

Anne was a brilliant and beautiful woman. William did not understand how anyone could be attracted to him. In time, they became "soul" mates." William loved her from the beginning of his ordeal, and for reasons that William could not explain, she was in love with him.

William proposed and married Anne. They chose to go on a honeymoon when his psychiatrist gave him the green light. William was on a leave of absence for 1 year to resolve his addiction problem, and when he returned to work, there was radical acceptance by those who knew his ordeal.

Suggested Reading

1. Berge KH, Seppala MD, Schipper AM. Chemical dependency and the physician. Mayo Clin Proc. 2009;84(7):625–31. https://doi.org/10.1016/S0025-6196(11)60751-9. PMID: 19567716. Review.
2. Chapoutot M, Peter-Derex L, Bastuji H, Leslie W, Schoendorff B, Heinzer R, Siclari F, Nicolas A, Lemoine P, Higgins S, Bourgeois A, Vallet GT, Anders R, Ounnoughene M, Spencer J, Meloni F, Putois B. Cognitive behavioral therapy and acceptance and commitment therapy for the discontinuation of long-term benzodiazepine use in insomnia and anxiety disorders. Int J Environ Res Public Health. 2021;18(19):10222. https://doi.org/10.3390/ijerph181910222. PMID: 34639523.

3. Day E, Daly C. Clinical management of alcohol withdrawal syndrome. Addiction. 2022;117(3):804–14. https://doi.org/10.1111/add.15647. Epub 2021 Aug 22. PMID: 34288186.
4. Fitzsimons MG, de Sousa GS, Galstyan A, Quintão VC, Simões CM. Prevention of drug diversion and substance use disorders among anesthesiologists: a narrative review. Braz J Anesthesiol. 2023;73(6):810–8. https://doi.org/10.1016/j.bjane.2023.07.008. Epub 2023 Jul 28. PMID: 37517585.
5. Ryan E, Hore K, Power JT. The relationship between physician burnout and depression, anxiety, suicidality and substance: a mixed methods and systematic review. Front Public Health. 2023;11:1133484. https://doi.org/10.3389/fpubh.2023.1133484. eCollection 2023. PMID: 37064688.
6. Silverstein JH, Silva DA, Iberti TJ. Opioid addiction in anesthesiology. Anesthesiology. 1993;79(2):354–75. https://doi.org/10.1097/00000542-199308.
7. Starks SM, Carroll Turpin MA, Reed BC, Grissom MO. Addiction medicine: benzodiazepine use disorder. FP Essent. 2024;546:16–22.

Amniotic Fluid Embolism

25

Chris Landry

A 25-year-old G1P0 patient was progressing well and comfortable in labor with an epidural in place. Her physical exam, prior to the epidural, showed a cervix 5 cm dilated, and the baby was at station 0. Her past medical history was noncontributory as well as a urine analysis that was negative for protein. The fetal heart rate was 120, and her rhythm strip revealed early decelerations, consistent with benign head compressions, which was reassuring. The examination, 60 min later, measured the cervix at 10 cm and plus one station.

The room was prepared for a vaginal delivery, and the patient was instructed to push. Chris made his way to the obstetrical floor with two visiting medical students. He was in the nursing office where the swipe board was hung and Chris was teaching FHR (fetal heart tracings).

After 30 min of pushing, the baby was born with an APGAR score of 9 after the first minute and 10 five minutes later. The husband and wife took turns holding the baby, and it was transparent that this was the most special moment in both of their lives. Twenty minutes later, the episiotomy was finished, and the patient returned to her room.

One hour later, with the mother holding the baby, she lost consciousness, and the baby was caught by the father, before hitting the floor. The mother was blue and the father screamed for help.

The initial vital signs of the mother were blood pressure 60/40, heart rate 30 beats/min, oxygen saturation—not measurable, and respiratory rate—0. The neurological exam was positive for fixed dilated pupils, absence of corneal reflexes, and no response to a painful stimulus.

Anesthesia was called stat, and the patient was intubated while the labor and delivery nurses performed CPR. A large-bore IV was placed to begin a pharmacological resuscitation. Chris and his students pushed the crash cart into the room. The AED was attached to the patient, and the patient was in ventricular fibrillation. Two hundred joules were delivered, and the patient became asystolic. After 1 mg of epinephrine, the heart remained asystolic. A second dose of epinephrine resulted in

C. Scher, *Anesthesia Conversations*,
https://doi.org/10.1007/978-3-032-05354-1_25

sinus tachycardia of 120 beats per minute. Chris felt the femoral artery, and there was a palpable pulse. The automated blood pressure device showed a BP of 55/25 and CPR was held.

"We need to know the pulmonary artery pressure. I can put in an introducer and a PA catheter in 10 minutes. Give me an Intro and I will float the Swan Ganz as long as there is adequate blood flow to the lungs. Lucas initiated a norepinephrine infusion at 10 micrograms per minute. Three minutes after the infusion began, the blood pressure was 70/40. The pulse oximeter was 78%. Chris did a rapid bronchoscopy, and his view was obscured by pink frothy foam. A sample of blood for an ABG was carried by Billy to the obstetrical ICU revealed a pH 6.9 Oxygen 39 CO_2-79 and Hct-19. The patient was not being ventilated nor oxygenated!"

The respiratory team arrived with a ventilator. They inspected the blood gas results and set up pressure control settings with a PEEP of 10 and FiO_2 of 100%. With a blood pressure of 82/43, Chris could not get the balloon to step up into the pulmonary artery. After 10 min, the Swan-Ganz Catheter entered the pulmonary artery. The PA pressure was 75 systolic. Leon asked for a TEE. He sent a resident to the cardiac operating room to wheel it down to the obstetrical ICU.

Leon was able to get the view that he wanted. The right ventricle was failing. The PA pressure was so elevated that the right ventricular ejection fraction was poor. The previous blood gas was now interpreted as severe pulmonary hypertension with right ventricular failure. The only treatment that could work is ECMO. The tech who sets up cardiopulmonary bypass and ECMO was still in the hospital. Chris wanted to talk to his students while at the same time trying to save a life. While rare, Chris made this scenario of a possible amniotic fluid embolism the topic of this learning clinical case.

"Amniotic fluid, fetal cells, hair, or other debris enters into the maternal pulmonary circulation, leading to cardiovascular collapse. The etiology largely remains unknown. It can also occur during an abortion, after abdominal trauma, and during an amnio-infusion. The prevailing teaching explanation addresses that is that a breach of the barrier between maternal blood and amniotic fluid forces the entry of amniotic fluid into the systemic circulation. This results in a physical obstruction of the pulmonary circulation. The presenting signs and symptoms of AFE involve many organ systems. Clinical signs and symptoms are acute dyspnea, cough, hypotension, cyanosis, fetal bradycardia, encephalopathy, acute pulmonary hypertension, and coagulopathy."

A cardiac surgeon responded to the stat page sent by the obstetrical service. "Start the Heparin! The desired ACT is 350–400." The first dose of heparin administered was 10,000 units in increments of 5000 units until he reached an ACT close to 400.

A continuous infusion of heparin was initiated. The tech chose venoarterial ECMO. She inserted one cannula into the right common femoral vein. The tip of the cannula is directed by fluoroscopy to the junction of the inferior vena cava and right atrium. This cannula is used for deoxygenated blood extraction. The left femoral and the right iliac arteries served to deliver oxygenated blood. After blood products were transfused, the ABG was normal, and the lactate was 7.

ECMO, blood products, and electrolyte management allowed the patient to have normal hemodynamics. Several attempts to weaning from ECMO failed. Above all, the patient's neurological status was improving. Renal and hepatic function were normalizing. The cardiac surgeon discussed with everyone in the ICU that the patient met the criteria for a right ventricular assist device.

The onset of pulmonary hypertension was abrupt in a young healthy patient. Those patients are part of a small cohort who could recover from severe pulmonary hypertension.

With inhaled nitric oxide and time, the patient was weaned off the RVAD after one month since the baby was born. Above all, her neurological status was normal, and she recovered 100%. With nutrition and physical therapy, she was discharged healthy with a rebirth of her lost faith.

Suggested Reading

1. Coggins AS, Gomez E, Sheffield JS. Pulmonary embolism and amniotic fluid embolism. Obstet Gynecol Clin North Am. 2022;49(3):439–60. https://doi.org/10.1016/j.ogc.2022.02.015. PMID: 36122978.
2. Nagarsheth NP, Pinney S, Bassily-Marcus A, Anyanwu A, Friedman L, Beilin Y. Successful placement of a right ventricular assist device for treatment of a presumed amniotic fluid embolism. Case reports. Anesth Analg. 2008;107(3):962–4.
3. Pacheco LD, Saade G, Hankins GD, Clark SL, Shamshirsaz AA. Amniotic fluid embolism. Obstet Gynecol Clin North Am. 2016;43(4):779–90. https://doi.org/10.1016/j.ogc.2016.07.001. PMID: 27816160.
4. Shamshirsaz AA, Clark SL. Amniotic fluid embolism. Obstet Gynecol Clin North Am. 2016;43(4):779–90. https://doi.org/10.1016/j.ogc.2016.07.001. PMID: 27816160.
5. Sparrow CT, LaRue SJ, Schilling JD. Intersection of pulmonary hypertension and right ventricular dysfunction in patients on left ventricular assist device support: is there a role for pulmonary vasodilators? Circ Heart Fail. 2018;11(1):e004255. https://doi.org/10.1161/CIRCHEARTFAILURE.117.004255.
6. Yu B, Ichinose F, Bloch DB, Zapol WM. Inhaled nitric oxide. Br J Pharmacol. 2019;176(2):246–55. https://doi.org/10.1111/bph.14512. Epub 2018 Nov 16. PMID: 30288739.

Complex Regional Pain Syndrome Type 1

26

Steve McEnroe

Steven MacEnroe is 63. His professional education included a BS and MD degree from LSU Baton Rouge, and an anesthesiology residency at Trinity, New Orleans. Steve grew up in the "Irish Channel." The area is bounded by Jackson Ave, Delachaise, Tchouopitoulas, and Magazine Street.

The area earned its name in the middle of the 1800s mass immigration from Ireland. St. Patrick's Day is like no other in the world and was the perfect reflection of those who lived in it. Rather than the usual beads tossed from Mardi Gras floats, cabbage and raw potatoes were thrown to the crowd like howitzers from those on the floats. The channel did not include any other culture other than the Irish.

Steven was ready to use his skills to take on the world by the end of his second year of a three-year residency. Steve was guaranteed a faculty position by the end of his CA-1 year. At the end of his CA-2 year, he enlisted in the Navy to go to Iraq.

The recruiter told Steve he would be working in a military hospital 25 miles from Baghdad. That plan never happened. Despite his protest, he was stationed on a Navy Huey-like helicopter to extract the wounded and start the first stage of resuscitation. Steve started an intravenous line to administer normal saline, pain meds, and antibiotics. The chopper usually landed in a hot zone, and Steven was trained to fight man-to-man if need be. Steven was in more firefights than he bargained for.

On the pickup of a wounded Marine, a bullet pierced through his right leg, just below the knee. He grabbed his leg, and it was still there. He grabbed a tourniquet out of his pack. It saved his life. Blood was transfused at the base hospital. There were no vascular injuries, but the tibia was shattered. The Navy put Steve on the next flight out to have surgery at Landstuhl Regional Medical Center in Germany.

Steve underwent a two-step approach to his injury. An external fixator stabilized the tibia, and two months later, a more definitive plating of the tibia would follow. Steve was grateful that he was alive, but the pain of his injury would agonize him for the rest of his life. His severe pain evolved to Complex Regional Pain Syndrome (CRPS) Type 2. (Type 1—there is no nerve injury; Type 2—this is a nerve injury.)

C. Scher, *Anesthesia Conversations*,
https://doi.org/10.1007/978-3-032-05354-1_26

Complex regional pain syndrome is a form of chronic pain that usually affects an arm or a leg. CRPS can develop as a result of an injury, surgery, stroke, or heart attack. The pain is out of proportion to the severity of the initial injury. Signs and symptoms of CRPS include: continuous burning or throbbing pain, sensitivity to touch or cold, swelling of the painful area, changes in skin temperature, alternating between sweat and cold, changes in skin color, ranging from white and blotchy to red or blue, changes in skin texture, thin or shiny skin, changes in hair and nail growth, joint stiffness, swelling, muscle spasms, tremors, and weakness. Many of these symptoms are irreversible.

Symptoms may change over time and vary from person to person. Pain, swelling, redness, noticeable changes in temperature, and hypersensitivity (particularly to cold and touch) usually occur first. Despite an early diagnosis, Steve, over time, had all of these changes. He tried every option and had mild relief from spinal cord stimulation, until he did not. He lost every inch of resolve left in his body and begged for an amputation.

Steve had multiple consultations. Only one surgeon agreed that amputation was necessary. Steve faced a dilemma of having a phantom limb or dealing with the torture of living with his CRPS-2.

The surgeon who agreed to amputate had a frank discussion, a discussion based on years of experience of the trade-off of CRPS for amputation. After five antidepressants, three atypical antipsychotic medications, several trials of narcotics, gabapentin, countless hours of psychiatry sessions and group therapy, he was done. To give himself peace of mind, the leg had to come off. He stood by his introspective and spiritual belief that his tortured soul would find peace of mind with the amputation. Booze kept the darkness at bay.

"Phantom limb pain occurs in 80 percent of amputees. 75% recover by two years and the current therapies are much more effective than they are for CRPS-2." Steve's new doctor wanted Steve to try group therapy targeted at life as an amputee.

The amputation was uneventful. There was not a moment of phantom limb pain. Unlike so many, the prosthesis was not a problem. Like so many of the soldiers who served, Steve's PTSD remained unaddressed. He had most of the symptoms of PTSD; panic attacks, insomnia, nightmares, with triggers that were all related to his tour in Iraq. Steve finally accepted psychotherapy and dialectical group therapy. There were so many like him. His PTSD never resolved, but his treatments taught him to live with it.

After an interview with Chris, Steve became Director of Trauma at Trinity. With his military experience and knowledge of CRPS and PTSD, Chris saw a dimension in Steve that added to the quality of the care of the trauma patient. His teaching talent was superior, and his impact on the development of the department was profound.

Suggested Reading

1. Bruehl S. Complex regional pain syndrome. BMJ. 2015;351:h2730. https://doi.org/10.1136/bmj.h2730. PMID: 26224572

2. Halicka M, Vittersø AD, Proulx MJ, Bultitude JH. Neuropsychological Changes in Complex Regional Pain Syndrome (CRPS). Behav Neurol. 2020;2020:4561831. https://doi.org/10.1155/2020/4561831. eCollection 2020. PMID: 32399082
3. Kaur A, Guan Y. Phantom limb pain: a literature review. Chin J Traumatol. 2018;21(6):366–8. https://doi.org/10.1016/j.cjtee.2018.04.006. Epub 2018 Dec 4. PMID: 30583983.
4. Rose E. Complex regional pain syndrome: diagnosis and management. Nurs Stand. 2023;38(4):57–61. https://doi.org/10.7748/ns.2023.e11968. Epub 2023 Mar 20. PMID: 36938711.
5. Tijsen LM, Derksen EW, Achterberg WP, Buijck BI. Challenging rehabilitation environment for older patients. Clin Interv Aging. 2019;14:1451–60. https://doi.org/10.2147/CIA.S207863. eCollection 2019. PMID: 31496672

27 Life After Leg Amputation

Tara Boston, Sofia Gangliano, Lily Tran, Lauren Garland, Whitney Jackson

As each 6 train approaches the 28th Street Station, the overhead loudspeaker always makes the same announcement that all passengers should wait behind the yellow line on the floor. If you are too close to the train and stick your head out to see the train coming, anything could happen. Most, if not all of the commuters, take a step back toward the wall of the station to avoid a slip onto the track or a push by some insane asshole who is going for the kill. There is a small cohort of riders who are suicidal and take a flying leap onto the track. Often, they are not successful and are almost mortally wounded. They spend months at Trinity Hospital, where the trauma team attempts to reconstruct their bodies.

Tara was always afraid that someone would grab her and toss her onto the coming train. She put her back on the back wall of the subway station and would not dare look down the tracks if the train was coming. The loudspeaker said that the 6 train was pulling up to the station, and "everyone should move back from the tracks," Tara was against the wall when two men with ski hats covering their faces grabbed her and tossed a screaming Tara onto the tracks of an incoming train. She jumped back from the tracks onto the platform. She was seconds too late back, and her right leg was sheared off by a 40-mile-per-hour train.

Tara could see her leg just above the knee, on the track. While screaming in pain, ten riders organized by a man with the words "Viet Nam Vet" on his cap, became a small militia" to save Tara. The Vet gave orders to this group of seven women and three men specific tasks to save Tara. 911 was called.

On the first inspection, her leg was the only part of her body injured. The Vet unbuckled his belt and wrapped it around her leg to serve as a tourniquet to the exposed and torn femoral artery. The belt slowed the hemorrhage down by approximately 50%, which was not enough. The father of a nine-year-old took his son's belt and tightened it above the first tourniquet. The Viet Nam Vet had already used his hand around the femoral artery to stop the bleeding.

The EMT had in their ambulance a surgical clamp, and the artery was fully clamped. Tara was awake and alert and "lost her mind" from the pain. She was

C. Scher, *Anesthesia Conversations*,
https://doi.org/10.1007/978-3-032-05354-1_27

white as a ghost from the blood loss. The EMT team called the trauma team at the hospital to fill a cooler with RBCs and FFP. The hematocrit of PRBCs is around 70, and the hematocrit of FFP is zero. Giving a unit of PRBCs and a bag of FFP would be the same as giving blood with a hematocrit of 35. Maintaining this ratio kept the hematocrit around 35.

The remaining leg was shredded, and there was no chance of replantation. Tara bypassed the emergency room and was taken by stretcher to operating room 11, which was always set up for a trauma. Tara's airway exam was normal, and a rapid sequence induction and intubation were uneventful. Sevoflurane was the basis of her anesthetic until her blood pressure "tanked." While the anesthesia team was waiting for the results of a blood gas, it was clear that more blood products were needed. Norepinephrine at 15 mcg a minute restored her blood pressure to a normal range. The pulse pressure from her arterial line normalized, and the transfusions stabilized her to a point that the norepinephrine was no longer needed. There was hemostasis on the remaining stump on her leg and liters of saline were pumped into the wound to wash it out. Three wound vacuums were bound to the stump, and closure could not be considered until the stump was clean and dry.

Tara underwent six surgeries in two years. She went from a wound infection to wound infections, no less than ten times. The site was periodically debrided to where it bled, assuring that there was enough flow of blood. The eventual final plan was to close the wound with alloderm and skin grafts. Alloderm is an acellular dermal matrix made of collagen, elastin, and laminin that is fabricated from human cadaver skin. The immediate plan consisted of daily debridements of devitalized tissue, washouts, and wound vacuums.

Tara thought that her stump issues were starting to migrate behind her. She was no longer embarrassed when her stump was seen in public. The next step was to fit her for a prosthesis. She envisioned a return to work, restoring a social life, and the true freedom to engage in the passions of her life. Her hopelessness had waned. With her phantom limb pain under control, she was more than ready to get back to work.

Tara chose her college and medical school solely based on price. She earned her B.S. at Hunter College. Her medical school and her anesthesia residency were at Downstate. Tara was street smart and only grew tougher working in New York's underserved hospitals. She developed coping skills that were transparent from the day she was injured. The prosthesis that promised so much hope developed into another jab at her punished life.

As usual with many patients who have a prosthesis, the stump over time shrinks and the prosthesis becomes painful. The skin of the stump started to look like a "bed sore." There were long periods of time that she had to heal and be refitted for another prosthesis. Tara suffered from back pain, poor balance, and an intense fear of falling. The prosthesis was exhausting as she walked in a manner to minimize her discomfort. By four o'clock in the afternoon, her day in the operating room had to end. Each day at work was an event.

Tara was able to compartmentalize her entire horrific event to get over the PTSD she developed. Above all, she needed to start fresh. Tara was ready to pack her bags and go to a city that could replace New York. Chicago, Boston, Philadelphia, Atlanta, and the Bay Area were on her list. It takes months of living in a city to judge if it is the right fit.

The American Society of Anesthesiology was in New Orleans at the same time that she had recovered enough to manage any task. Her prosthesis was comfortable, and the limp was, for the most part, gone. Her PTSD was in the past, and her body image was restored to the way she remembered it.

After her first lunch, while looking at the exhibits, two women came over and introduced themselves. Sofia and Lily asked Tara if she had any dinner plans. Tara was aghast. Who are these girls? They both had an ASA badge with their names. They were M.D.s. They had Mardi Gras beads around their necks. They were both fashionably dressed, wearing clothes from the most notable designers. Above all, they seemed "fun."

"There are thousands of people at this meeting! Why and how did you pick me? You do not even know me!"

"We are part of a new, growing Department of Anesthesia in New Orleans at Trinity Hospital. We are both Associate Professors at Trinity School of Medicine. Lily is the Program Director. I was one of the cardiac anesthesia attendings who sat next to you during the morning session on cardiac anesthesia."

You asked two questions at the end of the session. Those questions were profound. I looked at your badge, and it had your name on it, but unlike all of the other badges, there was no indication of where you were from. I went to the membership desk and looked up your name. This is all very legal. I saw that you were from New York City.

"We are recruiting to build our new department. If you ever consider living away from New York City, we can show you why New Orleans might be a great fit. If you are interested in a total immersion into New Orleans and our department, I would love to take you around New Orleans and our Department at Trinity. No worries, no pressure. We get how you could be suspicious with this approach. If this does not work for you, I am sure you will say that at least he had fun together."

"I never turn down fun, so sure, I'm in! When do we start?"

"It is four o'clock now. If you have no plans we can start in five minutes!"

Sofia was the self-appointed Director of Social Events. "Tara, coffee or something stronger?"

"Of course, something stronger or better said, much stronger."

Sofia started to text furiously. She invited Laura Garland and Whitney Jackson to join them at the bar at The Four Seasons, New Orleans. Whitney and Laura were both African Americans who were born and raised in New Orleans. They joined the Department about six months ago. Sofia wanted Tara to see black women since the faculty had more women than men and more people of color than not. Sofia thought that the demographics of the department would be its best selling point.

The bar was stunning. Sophia recommended that the drinks were inherent to New Orleans. Tara wanted to follow each suggestion and joined everyone in choosing the Sazerac. Sofhia was being Sofia. She was always "out there" and warmed up

Tara with her lude jokes and animated conversation. After thirty minutes, Sofhia called United Cab. The next stop was "Baroness on Baronne."

The Baroness was an African American bar. Sofia wanted to show Tara fun in a city with a thriving African American presence.. This time it was the Ramos Gin Fizz. Although it was only six PM, the place was hopping. Sofia's plan was working. The music was 80s funk, and the Atomic Dog had everyone singing. Tara grew up with her parents' music. While it was way too early for dancing, Laura and Whitney danced with others on the empty dance floor.

"Tara, you will find an itinerary online that will be posted by the time you get back to the hotel. Essentially you will meet several Department Chairs, have a tour of all anesthetizing locations, meet several departmental Chairs, lunch with residents and interviews with three attendings and the Chief Resident. Chris will be the last stop. Is it possible to discuss a case or two with the residents at lunch? Pick any case you want to discuss; a case that you have had that is academically interesting."

Tara dug deep down in her mind. The lecture about perioperative medications was easy and funny. Chris was in the audience. He joined the women for the excursion around the city.

"There is always confusion about a patient's medications; what to give and what to hold. Decisions are made from guidelines. Guidelines are made in a conference room by people who might be in the know of the medications. It is based on facts and personal experiences. I will discuss those that are most controversial. Here is where we stand today. The list is practical and we will go through the list."

Tara did not have a touch of stage fright during her presentation. She was relaxed, funny, and very informative. Chris was in the audience. He made up his mind to do whatever it takes to recruit her.

Suggested Reading

1. Esquenazi A. Gait analysis in lower-limb amputation and prosthetic rehabilitation. Phys Med Rehabil Clin N Am. 2014;25(1):153–67. https://doi.org/10.1016/j.pmr.2013.09.006. PMID: 24287245.
2. Isaacs-Itua A, Sedki I. Management of lower limb amputations. Br J Hosp Med (Lond). 2018;79(4):205–10. https://doi.org/10.12968/hmed.2018.79.4.205. PMID: 2962098. Review.
3. Paniagua AR, Mundy LR, Klassen A, Biswas S, Hollenbeck ST, Pusic AL, Gage MJ. Resilience through practicing acceptance: a qualitative study of how patients cope with the psychosocial experiences following limb-threatening lower extremity trauma. J Plast Reconstr Aesthet Surg. 2022;75(10):3722–31. https://doi.org/10.1016/j.bjps.2022.06.022. Epub 2022 Jun 18. PMID: 36089472.
4. Sinha R, van den Heuvel WJ, Arokiasamy P, van Dijk JP. Influence of adjustments to amputation and artificial limb on quality of life in patients following lower limb amputation. Int J Rehabil Res. 2014;37(1):74–9. https://doi.org/10.1097/MRR.0000000000000038. PMID: 2415786.
5. Ülger Ö, Yıldırım Şahan T, Çelik SE. A systematic literature review of physiotherapy and rehabilitation approaches to lower-limb amputation. Physiother Theory Pract. 2018;34(11):821–34. https://doi.org/10.1080/09593985.2018.1425938.

28 Failed Back Syndrome

John Caruso

"Johnny" Caruso's hubris was unwavering when asked where he was from. He was from Manhattan, the borough of New York that people are most familiar with. He did not elaborate on Manhattan. If someone knew nothing about Manhattan, it was just too exhausting to explain. There was New York City and the rest, the United States.

John loved Hunter College. He was an English major, and his GPA and MCAT put him up there with the best medical school applicants in the country. He was offered ten interviews and was a no-show for nine of them. What seemed crazy, John wanted to go to Bologna, Italy. He did not care if it was a six-year medical school.

His family had a successful flatware and cutlery business for a century. The first store was in Bologna. The family had 20 stores in Western Europe, and his parents wanted him to be a physician, but Johnny wanted in on the family business. He wanted to live in Italy to be near the center of the family business. When asked if he truly wanted to go to medical school in Italy, he always responded, "I will give it a shot !"

Johnny took his time to complete the 6-year program. It took him 8 years. He spent 2 years working at the family's main store. Without a single rotation in anesthesiology, he applied for a residency in the field. He summed it up with "easy job, excellent financial rewards." After 8 years, he didn't give a shit about any field of medicine. All of his thoughts about practicing medicine were far from firm.

Johnny applied to 50 anesthesia programs. He was offered four interviews: UIC, Temple, University of Maryland, and Trinity. Because he was a foreign medical school graduate, his mentor from Hunter encouraged him to apply to a different specialty that was not so competitive.

Johnny's manner in a conversation was unique. His time in the family store transformed him into a conversationalist who could capture anyone's attention. Johnny Caruso's manner was perfect at his interviews.

Lily was impressed with his application. The three other faculty members were in agreement with Lily. They were all concerned that their online website would

C. Scher, *Anesthesia Conversations*,
https://doi.org/10.1007/978-3-032-05354-1_28

have a student from Bologna. Johnny Caruso, on the website, signaled that the Trinity anesthesia residency had to go deep on their match list to get anyone. John was a PR nightmare and said yes when asked if they could take his name off the website.

"Chris, I do not get it! He has become an excellent resident." "He was a fuck up in Italy and now outworks anyone and has the highest scores on our department tests." Lily was sure that she was missing something. Somewhere down the line, the puzzle piece that made Johnny a star would be discovered.

Midway through his CA-2 year, Johnny was exhausted and depressed with the all-nighters from trauma. The 2 AM epidurals for laboring patients, preoperative consults, and the tedium of doing three hysterectomies in a row exhausted John. He evolved to feeling bored.

Johnny was the perfect team player who always followed the chain of command. He kept his emotions close to his heart and wanted out of anesthesia. A pain management fellowship would be aligned with his entrepreneurial trait in the family. He completed his one-year fellowship in pain management at the Tulane School of Medicine.. He was on a path that put him on the money track.

Johnny worked with his father to create his business model for a pain center. His business model would include a pain doctor, psychologist, psychiatrist, social workers, and a nutritionist. The overhead in Manhattan was enormous. The office space plus essential items: fluoroscopy, ultrasound, X-ray, and staff was close to 20,000 a month. The overhead in Jefferson Parish, just outside of New Orleans, was 1/3 of that in New York.

Johnny's plan was to initially keep the overhead down while generating a long list of chronic pain patients. He would do acute pain one day a week in the hospital and four days a week for chronic pain targeted at his self-made niche of patients with "failed back syndrome." He hired a public relations group to market his niche. There would be no negatives in his business model. He would not have any part in making chronic pain patients addicts from narcotic prescriptions in exchange for expensive nerve blocks.

A 57-year-old male from Harahan had a history of work-related back pain (construction worker) with right radicular pain. His insurance required a trial of three epidural steroid injections before the simple removal of a herniated disc at L3L4. The herniated nucleus pulposus releases cytokines and other mediators of inflammation that result in a radiculitis. Elevated levels of phospholipase A2, interleukin 6 and 8, and TNF-alpha are inflammatory markers that react with the spinal nerve roots to cause severe pain. Steroids have an anti-inflammatory effect by decreasing phospholipase A and may block the transmission of C fibers. If helpful, epidural steroid relief lasts for only 3 months. The literature on epidural is ongoing, and its efficacy has always been in question for many years. It was a Medicare mandate that a trial of three epidurals must be performed prior to a surgical intervention.

The transforaminal approach deposits epidural steroids into the anterolateral epidural space where the herniated disc is located. This approach may be more effective than the midline approach. The duration, however, is similar to the midline approach. If the first injection does not work, a second transforaminal injection might work.

There remains a worldwide epidemic of failed back syndrome due to more senior patients living longer. Johnny did a comprehensive history and physical. He wanted to rule out organic diseases that caused back pain. Bloods were sent out: ESR, C-reactive protein, metabolic panel, creatine kinase, serum aldolase, ANA, and imaging. An order was put in for an MRI of the entire spine and a CT scan of the abdomen (pancreatic and renal cell cancer could cause back pain). Within the confines of the Johnny's pain center, there was an office for a psychiatrist. The money generated by the psychiatrist was only for the psychiatrist. The office space for the psychiatrist was free. Between mood disorders, addiction, and general psychiatry, it was the dream job for most psychiatrists. No overhead at all.

A 55-year-old construction worker had an appointment for an increasing pain score in his back over the last year. He was prescribed hydrocodone, diclofenac, and neurontin after a visit to the emergency room. Prior to discharge, an appointment was made for the following day with Dr. Caruso.

Imaging does not always give the answer. It did in this case. The flexion-extension films revealed that vertebral bodies at L3L4 were bone-on-bone and sliding (anterolisthesis). There was a loss of height (L3L4) and severe osteoarthritis. At L4L5, there was a desiccated disc bone-on-bone and sliding forward. The MRI revealed moderate bilateral foraminal narrowing at both L3L4 and L4 L5. Moderate foraminal stenosis is usually asymptomatic. Essentially, the cause of back pain was clear: severe osteoarthritis of the entire spine, sliding vertebral bodies L4L5, and severe spinal stenosis at L4L5. The cervical spine showed severe osteoarthritis but no spinal stenosis, and all discs were intact. There were T2 signals on MRI at both L3L4 and L4L5. The degenerative changes affect the integrity of the spinal cord and are T2 signals on the spinal cord.

Johnny recommended a lumbar spinal fusion. He consulted Dr. Manganini, a well-known neurosurgeon, who agreed with Johnny.

A two-level fusion that involves removing the intervertebral discs between the vertebrae and replacing them with a bone graft. Rods, screws, and or plates are placed until the bone graft heals. The patient has to be well enough and strong enough to endure the tribulations of the whole process. John agreed with the surgical plan, and his case proceeded without complications.

The ongoing degeneration of the remainder of the spine could occur later in his life and need further surgery. Ongoing spinal degeneration could lead to pain at the original level of surgery if he does not respond to conservative treatment, including medications. With any back surgery, scar tissue could impact the nerves, which would require a second and third opinion.

Multiple studies have shown that the back pain caused by foraminal stenosis is associated with greater rates of FBSS (Failed Back Syndrome) than pain caused by recurrent disc herniation. Entrapment of the superior cluneal nerve is an often-overlooked diagnosis in patients presenting with lower back pain. The cluneal nerve functions as purely sensory nerves, and the superior cluneal nerve and the middle cluneal nerve provide cutaneous innervation to the buttock and posterior presacral region.

The neurosurgeons and orthopedic surgeons wanted Johnny to manage the pain in all spine surgeries. Johnny was pleased to get the work during a time when he was first starting his pain center. He needed the work. It could take a year before he had a cohort of failed back cases to turn a profit.

Johnny was not a fan of PCA. The patients had moments of being pain-free followed by moments of severe pain. The patients initially went with the flow but panicked when there was no sustainable relief. When the pump was interrogated each morning. The number of attempts versus pain relief was always problematic. Sixty attempts at a specific epoch often revealed 60 or more attempts, signaling panic. Dosing PCA is challenging. How do you set up a PCA with a heroin addict or simply a narcotic-tolerant patient?

Johnny managed the pain of those who were discharged. His regimen was oxycodone or hydrocodone, neurontin, acetaminophen, and valium for muscle spasms. Patients would be permitted to take NSAIDS at the four-week mark. There is some evidence that NSAIDS prevent the bone graft from healing. He called all of his patients at 7 AM and 4 PM and made an adjustment as needed. The goal was to prescribe narcotics for no longer than 4 weeks if possible.

After 6 months of relative comfort, lumbar pain returned. Johnny ordered an MRI. The list of possibilities was exhaustive. Did another level of his lumbar spine or thoracic disc become a problem? Was this a case of painful hardware? Did the dreaded severe spinal stenosis come into fruition at other levels? Did scarring affect the nerves from the first surgery?

Failed back surgery syndrome (FBSS) is defined by the International Association for the Study of Pain as lumbar spinal pain of unknown origin either persisting despite surgical intervention or appearing after surgical intervention for spinal pain originally in the same lumbar location. The pain may originate after surgery, or the surgery may exacerbate or insufficiently ameliorate existing pain.

The pathophysiology of failed back surgery syndrome is complex and is attributable to several possible factors. Lateral stenosis of the foramina is the most common structural cause. Pathologies in failed back surgery syndrome include painful disc degeneration, disc herniation, neuropathic pain, and pseudoarthrosis. Pathophysiological findings associated with FBSS and attributable to surgery include epidural fibrosis, increased spinal instability due to discectomy or laminectomy, and redistribution of load to adjacent disc tissue.

Psychosocial factors have been shown to have the strongest association with the development of failed back syndrome, which suggests that conservative treatments should be attempted first: spinal cord stimulation, gabapentin, antidepressants, physical therapy, and nerve blocks. Surgery is effective only if there is something seen on imaging that is believed to be the cause.

A second MRI demonstrated that the bone graft did not heal. There is a certain amount of doubt in the business of pain management. Johnny repeated his history and physical: The patient was a smoker and used NSAIDs. Nicotine disrupts the flow to a bone graft. Although not diagnosed, Johnny did not review his metabolic panel which revealed a blood sugar of 345. He had a BMI of 35, which caused a loading on the graft. Other medications that inhibit bone graft healing include steroids, proton pump inhibitors, certain chemotherapies, SSRI antidepressants, certain anticonvulsants, and bisphosphonates (for osteoporosis).

The plan was to place a new bone graft. He had to stop smoking for four weeks before the new bone graft and four weeks after the bone graft. BMPs could be used to stimulate bone growth. BMPs are "bone morphogenetic proteins." Bone morphogenetic proteins have been in use in spinal surgery since 2002. These proteins are members of the TGF-beta superfamily and guide mesenchymal stem cells to differentiate into osteoblasts to form bone in targeted tissues. These proteins are in all human bodies. They can be synthetic and concentrated for placement in the surgical area. The BMPs would hasten fusion.

Johnny had a massive evolution going on in his brain. Johnny's unacceptable successful cure rate only increased his resolve. He enjoyed his role as a healer. He had become passionate about his care for his cases and less about business. He became wealthy with the "new Johnny." His essential emotions added time for each patient and were no longer part of his business plan.

Suggested Reading

1. Alizadeh R, Sharifzadeh SR. Pathogenesis, etiology, and treatment of failed back surgery syndrome. Neurochirurgie. 2022;68(4):426–31. https://doi.org/10.1016/j.neuchi.2021.09.005. Epub 2021 Sep 17. PMID: 34543614 Review.
2. Amirdelfan K, Webster L, Poree L, Sukul V, McRoberts P. Treatment options for failed back surgery syndrome patients with refractory chronic pain: an evidence based approach. Spine (Phila Pa 1976). 2017;42(Suppl 14):S41–52. https://doi.org/10.1097/BRS.0000000000002217.
3. Chen YC, Lee CY, Chen SJ. Narcotic addiction in failed back surgery syndrome. Cell Transplant. 2019;28(3):239–47. https://doi.org/10.1177/0963689718796072. Epub 2018 Aug 31. PMID: 30168351.
4. Clancy C, Quinn A, Wilson F. The aetiologies of failed back surgery syndrome: a systematic review. J Back Musculoskelet Rehabil. 2017;30(3):395–402.
5. Danielle JR, Osti OL. Failed back surgery syndrome: a review article. Asian Spine J. 2018;12(2):372–9.
6. Miekiwiak G. Failed back surgery syndrome: no longer a surgeon's defeat – a narrative review. Medicina (Kaunas). 2023;59(7):1255. https://doi.org/10.3390/medicina59071255. PMID: 37512066.
7. Sebaaly A, Lahoud MJ, Rizkallah M, Kreichati G, Kharrat K. Etiology, evaluation, and treatment of failed back surgery syndrome. Asian Spine J. 2018;12(3):574–85.

The Celiac Plexus Block

29

Diana Lee

Ten years ago, Diana Lee's father, Minh, died of pancreatic cancer. Without any symptoms, he woke up one morning and noticed that the sclera of his eyes was yellow. His wife noticed that his entire body had a shade of yellow. Minh had not revealed to anyone in his family that he had boring pain in his back, diarrhea every day, and a slow but steady weight loss. As a medical examiner in the District of Columbia, he knew that he had pancreatic cancer for several weeks. The pancreatic cancer team at Memorial Sloan Kettering examined him two weeks before his wife noticed he was jaundiced. CT, MRI, and blood tests confirmed that he had Stage 4 pancreatic cancer. There was a heavy tumor load in his liver. He knew that he would not survive.

There were several clinical trials that developed during the Covid years. The messenger RNA science led to a vaccine that activates the immune system to recognize pancreatic cancer cells. Investigators needed to know if this technology would be efficacious. Stage 4 patients were not eligible for the "vaccine." If included, it would be difficult to determine efficacy when these patients could not be saved, and the data would be skewed away from the vaccine.

Minh's goal was to examine hundreds of clinical trials with the guidance of the team at Sloan Kettering, and most were at an early stage where definitive conclusions could not be found. His goal was to die without suffering. That was more than a tall order.

A stent in the biliary duct relieved his jaundice. He was at the point where the dose of opioids needed regular escalations. He was not dying comfortably. He wanted a celiac plexus block. If that did not work, he would go into hospice at home and overdose on his pills.

Diana grew up in Jackson, Mississippi, and was educated in the public-school system. She was an excellent student as a result of the combination of her intellect and work ethics. Her erudition was clearly the result of intense parenting with the highest level of supervision that was just short of oppression. Diane was accepted to the University of Mississippi (Ole Miss). She received a scholarship, making it the

C. Scher, *Anesthesia Conversations*,
https://doi.org/10.1007/978-3-032-05354-1_29

logical choice for a family with small means. Graduating cum laude was not enough to guarantee a spot in any medical school.

Most medical schools require community service. This was a must and could not be political, or simply trying to make an impression on a CV. While not "community service," Diana enrolled in USC's online Master of Public Health (MPH) concentration in Biostatistics and Epidemiology. While not community service, it seemed a perfect way to elevate her skill level in information that was essential for any physician, Diana completed the one-year Master's in her senior year.

The Master's program was a home run. She was accepted to Johns Hopkins School of Medicine and completed her anesthesiology residency and a pain fellowship at Hopkins. The experience with her father's pain inspired her to enter a pain management fellowship at her second home, Johns Hopkins. Diana chose pain management to help people through life. She wanted to be a healer, and pain management fit her just right with her specific niche being pancreatic cancer pain.

Pain from pancreatitis and pancreatic cancer is unrelenting, and the celiac plexus block is the most efficacious for both pancreatic pain from pancreatitis and pancreatic cancer. When the block did not work, it was always a deficiency in the block technique. Over time, the procedure and success rate have increased dramatically.

The celiac plexus is the largest plexus of the sympathetic nervous system. It contains preganglionic sympathetic fibers from greater and lesser splanchnic nerves as well as postganglionic sympathetic and preganglionic parasympathetic fibers. It provides sensory innervation and sympathetic outflow to the stomach, liver, spleen, pancreas, kidney, and GI tract up to the splenic flexure. Plexus is located at the level of T12-L2 (usually L1) and is anterior to the aorta in the retroperitoneal space. The classical method of the celiac plexus block has a failure rate of up to 30% of patients.

The block is often done by gastroenterologists with an upper GI endoscopy combined with ultrasound. A needle is passed through the stomach to the ultrasound image of the celiac plexus. This technique, over the last few years, has been proven to be more successful and safer than the old standard transabdominal blocks with fluoroscopy. Only patients with pancreatitis or pancreatic cancer were eligible for the endoscopic approach to the celiac plexus. Serious complications from a celiac plexus block and celiac plexus neurolysis are rare. The most frequent adverse events are diarrhea, orthostatic hypotension, and a transient increase in abdominal pain. The neurolytic block lasts 3–6 months.

Diana wanted to learn the endoscopic approach that was now "owned" by gastroenterologists. The Department of Gastroenterology agreed to allow Diana to train to use an endoscopic ultrasound approach to the block. Although a bit clumsy at first navigating the endoscope, she had identified the components of the ultrasound which is on the tip of the scope.

She was taught to troubleshoot if there were image problems with the scope or ultrasound. Once she was comfortable with the scope and the ultrasound images, the celiac plexus was easy to identify. A needle (27-gauge) was passed through the wall of the stomach, and absolute alcohol (ethanol) was injected around the plexus. If the location is correct, most patients will have a reduction of symptoms.

Diana had seen complications over time that she had seen but were well known and were amenable to treatment. With her technique of using an endoscopy and ultrasound, serious complications were not common, if not rare. Orthostatic hypotension and diarrhea secondary to blockade of sympathetic fibers comprised the most common and were easily treated adverse events. Less common complications including paraplegia (from damage to the artery of Adamkiewicz), local, spinal, or epidural injection, aortic or vena cava puncture and bleeding, and visceral organ injury were well described, but Diana had not encountered them.

She preferred to keep patients for 4 h in the PACU after the block. It was a moot point since most of the patients were already inpatients for to severe pain management and other complications related to pancreatic cancer.

Diana's goal was to develop a national and international reputation for pain management of pancreatic cancer. The volume of patients in severe pain grew by the day. While it was generally not accepted to do a prophylactic celiac plexus block, she agreed, but she did think the relatively safe block should be started once narcotics were prescribed. There was a sentiment that Diana was "blocking for bucks." Diana was horrified by people who thought that a trial of narcotics should be first. Diana wondered what the cutoff was for prescribing narcotics before she was needed.

"Was it a week of narcotics with nausea, break through pain, opioid induced hyperalgesia, itching, addiction, and delirium?" Was it two weeks with crescendo pain but a score that went from 4 to 7. There is a consensus that the block is extreme and conservative therapy should be first. Really?"

The architects for Trinity had a model for 10 procedure rooms for the gastroenterologists. Chris helped design a room for complicated procedures: esophageal stents, ERCPs, biliary stents, and gall retrievals. Diana's patients would be treated in this room. There are bariatric patients who can "eat through" a sleeve gastrectomy or gastric bypass. With an EGD, the gastroenterologists can sew across the lumen to make it smaller.

Diana Lee wanted exposure. They needed to be "advertised" that Diana was only treating exclusively pancreatic pain. She quickly arrived on the lecture circuit.

Chris had his first recruiting challenge. Was it possible to recruit anyone who was a Johns Hopkins lifer to come to a rebuilding city with a rebuilding hospital and a rebuilding anesthesia department? He could offer her a salary and time off that was double what she was receiving now. He could offer her a Master's at 36,000 a year and a Phd at 100,000 dollars a year. She would be nonclinical for 180 days to work/ per year to work on her projects and vacations. Chris thought it was an incredible offer.

Every New Orleanian anesthesiologist was a member of the New Orleans Anesthesia Society (NOAS). The cost of membership was 200 dollars a year. They met monthly at an event space in the Hotel Monteleone on Royal Street. On their website was the menu for the next meeting, the speaker, and the time. There was always an hour for cocktails. The evening cost 100 bucks including an open bar for the entire event. It evolved from an academic event to a 100% night out having fun. Chris invited Diana to speak at the NOAS and to stay in New Orleans as long as she wanted. This all-inclusive endeavor was free, from the taxi to pick her up at her home to the taxi to bring her home from the airport.

Chris sent the email at 8 AM Baltimore time. Diana responded 10 min later that she would come to the next Society meeting. Chris sent her an extensive email about the condition of New Orleans and its healthcare crisis. The only important information was the time of day and date she wanted to come. Chris wanted her to come the day before the meeting. That is when he could give her the hard sell.

Suggested Reading

1. Coveler AL, Mizrahi J, Eastman B, Apisarnthanarax SJ, Dalal S, McNearney T, Pant S, Precision Promise Consortium. Pancreas cancer-associated pain management. Oncologist. 2021;26(6):e971–82. https://doi.org/10.1002/onco.13796. Epub 2021 May 12. PMID: 33885205.
2. Lohse I, Brothers SP. Pathogenesis and treatment of pancreatic cancer related pain. Anticancer Res. 2020;40(4):1789–96. https://doi.org/10.21873/anticancer.14133. PMID: 32234867 Free PMC article. Review.
3. Rahman M, Washington L. The seemingly innocuous presentation of metastatic pancreatic tail cancer: a case report. J Med Case Rep. 2019;13(1):178. https://doi.org/10.1186/s13256-019-2125-5.
4. Strand DS, Law RJ, Yang D, Elmunzer BJ. AGA clinical practice update on the endoscopic approach to recurrent and acute and chronic pancreatitis. Gastroenterology. 2022;163(4):1107–14. https://doi.org/10.1053/j.gastro.2022.07.079. Epub 2022 Aug 22. PMID: 36008176 Review.
5. Yasuda I, Wang HP. Endoscopic ultrasound-guided celiac plexus block and neurolysis. Dig Endosc. 2017;29(4):455–62. https://doi.org/10.1111/den.12824. Epub 2017 Mar 9. PMID: 28160344 Review.

Treacherous Bariatric Surgery for an Anesthesiologist

30

Sydney Grossman, Laura Garland, James Murray

As far back as anyone who knew Sydney, he was a victim of child abuse. His parents did nothing for the health of their son. When Sydney was in the fifth grade, he was 220 pounds. He was front and center of most of the jokes by most children who are basically mean. He came to the emergency room with a fever and a rash, and the diagnoses were 1. influenza and 2. child abuse.

The pediatrician in the emergency room called child protective services, and Sydney was taken from his parents and put in a foster home. Most of the families who were interested in adopting an older child went through the foster home system. Because of Sydney's weight, most families declined to take Sydney when they saw his picture. After 10 months of waiting, Sydney was accepted into a home in St. Tammany Parish. The Kendall family took Sydney into their home.

Tom Kendall reached out to a child psychiatrist for guidance in Sydney's care. The psychiatrist recommended a general pediatrician, a nutritionist, a personal trainer, and a school that had a special education class. It was very credible that Sydney was diagnosed with a learning disorder; he was sick most of his life and abused by his family. The Kendalls took him on as a son as well as a project. His original parents never tried to get him back and they did everything possible to live as far away from Louisiana.

By the first year of high school, his BMI improved to 52 (68 inches, 354 pounds). His exercise tolerance and school grades improved. He tested out of special education and found a social network that accepted him. The hours of mental health care fixed what seemed to be broken, but made little headway with his food addiction.

Sydney was a stress eater and recognized that, but could not stop himself. He was on psych meds, engaged in therapy weekly, ate a better diet, but could not pass a vending machine without putting money into it.

By the age of 16, Sydney was diagnosed with metabolic syndrome: hypertension, diabetes, elevated triglycerides, elevated LDL, and fat in the waist. Metformin, a statin, and losartan were prescribed. His pediatrician noted that Sydney was diaphoretic and mildly tachypneic in the sitting position. Sydney said he had always

C. Scher, *Anesthesia Conversations*,
https://doi.org/10.1007/978-3-032-05354-1_30

been that way for many years. A pediatric cardiologist was consulted, and after a chest X-ray and transthoracic echocardiogram, bilateral fluffy infiltrates were visualized, and the ejection fraction on ECHO was 30%. Sydney had congestive heart failure. His blood pressure was 165/90. The hemoglobin A1C was 10.

A surgical consultant for bariatric surgery was ordered to discuss bariatric surgery at such a young age. After their consultation, a meeting was arranged to talk to the Kendalls after Sydney was medically optimized. Sydney was prescribed insulin for his diabetes and weight loss, captopril for hypertension, and Inderal for heart failure. An appointment was made after 2 weeks of medical therapy with the cardiologists.

Sydney was compliant with his medication. His hemoglobin A1C was down to 8, and his blood pressure was 143/80. The echocardiogram demonstrated an ejection fraction of 52% which was a marked improvement. It was time to meet the bariatric team. The surgery choices offered included a gastric bypass, sleeve gastrectomy, or a laparoscopic band.

The choice was made with uniform consensus. Sydney would have the gastric sleeve. He was too young to coexist with the physiologic derangements of a bypass. Surgery was actually the easiest part of the weight loss program. Sydney would need a 100% change in his approach to food. Family support is essential.

Sydney had to understand that he may never have a steak again. His sleeve would result in rapid weight loss, but Sydney's diet would significantly change as his new smaller stomach would not allow certain foods to pass.

The anesthesiologists thought a supervised diet and exercise over time would make this situation safer. Internal medicine and anesthesiologists agreed that his case should be postponed until he lost weight. There was no amount of weight loss that was a metric. Losing 25 lbs on a liquid diet would be a start. The purpose of the liquid diet was to remove the fat in the liver. The case was postponed for a month for a re-evaluation.

Anesthesiologists like challenges, but no anesthesiologist volunteered to do the case. Sydney regressed and ballooned up to 407 lbs. He could not lie flat without becoming short of breath. His air hunger was followed by sleep apnea. He "failed" the airway exam. Jimmy Murray and Laura Garland agreed, with hesitancy to do the case.

Sydney was a Mallampati four with an enormous neck that prevented a normal range of motion, protruding teeth, a recession of the lower mandible, and a thyromental distance that was normal.

As predicted, securing intravenous access with ultrasound guidance was necessary for both IVs. The second IV was a must. If one IV "went down: with no second IV," the case could become catastrophic. An arterial line was preferred for blood pressure management as it was unlikely that even a large cuff may not cover the arm. The blood pressures obtained in the clinic were done on the forearm which is not ideal.

Bariatric patients usually stay one night for pain control and to evaluate for a leak. Sydney was admitted to the surgical ICU for pain management, respiratory complications, any issues that may arrive like postoperative nausea and vomiting, and apnea.

The procedure chosen was for an awake intubation with a McGrath videoscope. With excellent nerve blocks and sedation, the McGrath was superior to a bronchoscope. Laura and James had the perfect conversation with Sydney to help him understand the airway process. He did understand that the dose for sedation could not be guaranteed due to his size. While awake, Sydney gargled three "cups" of prepackaged viscous lidocaine. He gargled each cup for as long as he could and then swallowed. The glossopharyngeal nerve was blocked.

James believed that a recurrent nerve block was risky but a must. The cricoid cartilage could not be found by palpation, but an ultrasound revealed an excellent image of his cricoid. The entire airway was anesthetized. with topical local anesthesia. An atomizer with 2% lidocaine was sprayed "just about everywhere". Small doses of midazolam were titrated until a total dose of 5 mg was achieved. Above all, a high flow nasal at 60 liters a minute preceded any sedation. Midazolam was chosen because it is readily reversed with flumazenil if the airway was lost. A tongue blade is rubbed around the hypopharynx to check the quality block. Sydney's airway was numb. He seemed alert but offered no complaints.

With awake intubation, the anesthesiologist has 10 min to work. By then, the local anesthetic is washed away with secretions. McGrath gave excellent exposure, but Sydney was biting hard on it. He became more agitated, and the view was lost.

"We need to redo the blocks," Jimmy. The recurrent laryngeal nerve is blocked from the underside of the vocal cords and into the trachea. It is blocked with a transtracheal puncture. The airway above the cords is captured by the internal branch of the superior laryngeal nerve. The nerves lie in the lateral corner of the epiglottis junction between the epiglottis and the tongue. An atomizer filled with local anesthetic is sprayed throughout the mouth that covers the glossopharyngeal and the internal branch of the superior laryngeal nerve from the upper side of the cords and up.

Alternatively, nerves of the airway can be blocked with a nebulizer filled with 2% lidocaine. You have to work fast as saliva will dilute the nebulized local anesthetic. An additional 2 mg of midazolam was titrated to effect, and Sydney was now cooperative for the McGrath. The endotracheal tube was passed with some struggle by Sydney. Once CO_2 was visualized on the monitor, Propofol was administered. A bronchoscope aided the exact desired depth. Any change of depth of the tube was performed with a fiberoptic scope inside the ETT to optimize its position. Would a generic MAC 4 laryngoscope work? Lauren and James would never know. If the patient had started to "fight back," airway sensation would be repeated with a smaller dose of lidocaine. Sydney's intubation was uneventful. In total, 250 mcg of Fentanyl, 100 mg of rocuronium, dexamethasone, and ondansetron were administered over the 60-minute case.

In the wee hours of the morning, Sydney had an abrupt change in his behavior. He had become frantic, aggressive, and was unresponsive to questions by the nursing staff. He did respond to pain when his right calf was pressed while restraints were being placed. A bedside ultrasound revealed a DVT in the right calf. When his hand was restrained, the pulse oximeter tone dropped, and the saturation displayed on the monitor was 84%. A non-rebreathing 100% oxygen mask was secured. A STAT CT-angio of his head and chest revealed a shower of pulmonary emboli and clots in his cerebral circulation. The decline of his mental status went along with the clots in his cerebral circulation.

The neurointerventional radiologists were called for an angiogram and clot retrieval. The anesthesia team had no problem with the induction and maintenance of general anesthesia. The plan was to essentially overdose Sydney with rocuronium and reverse with Bridion to allow a proper neurological assessment after the procedure was completed.

The entry point was the right femoral vein. The Seldinger technique was adapted by placing a catheter over a wire into the vein with fluoroscopic guidance. Multiple clots were retrieved from cerebral arteries. The interventional radiologists placed an IVC filter at the end of the neurointerventional intervention. A post-procedure CT scan did not reveal a brain that was hypoxic from the stroke.

Sydney went back from the CT scan to the Neurointerventional room for the extubation. The CT scan room had no airway equipment if there was an airway crisis after extubation. Everything that would be needed in an airway emergency was back in the neuro-suite. While the neurointerventional fellow wanted Sydney to be extubated in the CT room, Jimmy and Lauren explained in an aggressive tone, that extubation in the CT scan broke the most important fundamental guidelines in anesthesiology.

Sydney lost 200 pounds in 18 months. He no longer had a learning disorder or metabolic syndrome, and he was on no medication. There were no lingering neurological issues, and he soared both academically and, of equal importance, socially.

Isabella was his girlfriend in his senior year of college. She married after Sydney graduated from the University of Michigan. There were concerns that he had swung in the opposite direction when he weighed 150 pounds. That was his target weight. Sydney attended medical school at the University of Michigan and did his anesthesia residency at the University of Illinois in Chicago. His wife attended the Northwestern School of Journalism and became an anchorwoman on a news station in New Orleans. She was also an author of four books related to the politics of New Orleans. Sydney became a lifer in the department of anesthesia at Trinity.

Suggested Reading

1. Birns J, Qureshi S, Chen R, Bhalla A. Endovascular stroke treatment. Eur J Intern Med. 2014;25(7):584–91. https://doi.org/10.1016/j.ejim.2014.06.025. Epub 2014 Jul 14. PMID: 25034389 Review.
2. Marshall RV, Haas PJ, Schweinfurth JM, Replogle WH. Outcomes in super obese patients. JAMA Otolaryngol Head Neck Surg. 2016;142(8):772–6. https://doi.org/10.1001/jamaoto.2016.1089. PMID: 27228561
3. Mechanick JI, Apovian C, Brethauer S, Garvey WT, Joffe AM, Kim J, Kushner RF, Lindquist R, Pessah-Pollack R, Seger J, Urman RD, Adams S, Cleek JB, Correa R, Figaro MK, Flanders K, Grams J, Hurley DL, Kothari S, Seger MV, Still CD. Clinical practice guidelines for the perioperative nutrition, metabolic, and nonsurgical support of patients undergoing bariatric

procedures – 2019 update: cosponsored by American Association of Clinical Endocrinologists/ American College of Endocrinology, the Obesity Society, American Society for Metabolic & Bariatric Surgery, Obesity Medicine Association, and American Society of Anesthesiologists – executive esummary. Endocr Pract. 2019;25(12):1346–59. https://doi.org/10.4158/GL-2019-0406. Epub 2019.

4. Quigley S, College J, Mukherjee S, Patel K. Bariatric surgery: a review of normal postoperative anatomy and complications. Clin Radiol. 2011;66(10):903–14. https://doi.org/10.1016/j.crad.2011.04.017. Epub 2011 Jul 23. PMID: 21783182.
5. Singla V, Aggarwal S, Garg H, Kashyap L, Shende DR, Agarwal S. Outcomes in super obese patients undergoing laparoscopic sleeve gastrectomy. J Laparoendosc Adv Surg Tech A. 2018;28(3):256–62. https://doi.org/10.1089/lap.2017.0536. Epub 2017 Nov 3. PMID: 29099314.

31 Lumbar Surgery Complicated by Ischemic Optic neuropathy and Blindness

Robert Chase, **Michael Moss**

Robert Chase attended St. Augustine High School in New Orleans. His time at St. Augustine centered around his expertise in basketball, and he was heavily recruited to play at LSU. "St. Aug" offered students a comprehensive educational experience, but Robert's desire to play was greater than his desire to learn. He was way too busy playing hoops. He was missing an opportunity to become educated. Robert averaged 20 points a game until the next class of players became members of the team. The new class of players was bigger and faster than he was. The handwriting was on the wall. His place on the team was on the bench.

Robert's parents were successful in turning the switch in his brain to embrace education. Becoming a physician was his parents' goal. Robert had no goals for his future. Robert needed mentoring apart from his parents. He was struggling with school, and his brother Jalen, who was 10 years older, made a realistic path for Robert to ease on slowly into academics.

Jalen was on the faculty at Tulane as an Assistant Professor of History. He knew how to teach and ignite students to find a passion. He started Robert with level 101 classes in English, History, Statistics, and Spanish. At the end of his first year of year as a normal, everyday student, his GPA. was 3.0; straight Bs. The next semester was biology and chemistry; only two classes. They would be a challenge for Robert. Jalen wondered if Robert had ADHD, which was masked by his devotion and single-minded direction to a life of basketball.

Jalen was not expecting Robert to earn a degree in four years. His plan for Robert was for five years. Jalen checked in with Robert every day. Jalen was becoming essential to developing Robert. Jalen taught the basics of introspection. It would lead to a passion in his life other than basketball. Jalen was adding courses that could make them premed, prelaw, or pre-teaching.

Robert "killed it." His productivity increased each day. His Bs were now becoming As. The path was doing well in premed courses. He struggled with Calculus and Physics, but kept the flame alive with a combined GPA of 3.4. It was not the GPA needed for medical school.

C. Scher, *Anesthesia Conversations*,
https://doi.org/10.1007/978-3-032-05354-1_31

Robert had one link to basketball. On Saturday afternoons, he played pickup basketball at the S.E. Mackey Center in Baton Rouge. The center was the home of the best basketball players who were not part of LSU. Most were 5–10 years out from high school. There were no referees, and the games were more than physical.

There was always a crowd of spectators, and Robert did not refrain from showboating. Your team stayed on the court as long as it was winning. "You lose. You're out!" Robert's team was dominating in the final minute of the last game, but Robert came crashing down on his back after blocking a shot. He could not get up. This was the worst pain in his life.

While none of the spectators or players knew what a pain score was, he was clearly a ten out of ten, where 0 is no pain and 10 is the worst imaginable pain. He could not move his legs!

When EMS arrived, he was placed on a spine board. A cervical collar was secured on his neck, followed by a mask of oxygen at eight liters per minute. An 18-gauge IV was placed in a large vein at the left antecubital fashion. The plan was to go for a MRI to checked Robert from head to toe.

The MRI revealed two vertebral body fractures at L3L4 and L4L5. There was T2 signaling of the spinal cord at L4L5. T2 signaling means spinal cord involvement with the fracture. A bilateral laminectomy and fusion was the indicated surgery.

For the next four hours, Robert was prone with his head on a prone pillow. The pillow provided a cushion and a mirror at the base of the pillow that enabled the anesthesiologist to visualize pressure on the eyes and lips. The visualization of the eyes was confirmed by Mike Moss, the attending anesthesiologist. The integrity of the spinal cord was monitored with evoked potentials. An arterial line was placed to allow the blood pressure to be elevated to maintain adequate perfusion of the spinal cord.

Robert was turned from prone to supine for wake-up and extubation. Moments after extubation, Robert woke up and moved all four extremities with strong and normal motions. The case was perfect, until there was a tragic finding. Robert could not see out of his right eye.

Robert was at risk in the prone position for vision loss. During that period of time, his intraocular pressure rose from hours of compression on his eyes. A normal intraocular pressure is 10–20 mmHg. Intraocular pressures higher than 21 mmHg pose a risk for glaucoma, detached retina, and postoperative vision loss. Postoperative vision loss in patients undergoing surgery in the prone position is generally related to one of two causes: ischemic optic neuropathy or central retinal artery occlusion. Dr. Moss blamed himself for having this outcome.

There were essential steps that were not taken in this case. The bed should have been in 5–10 degrees reverse Trendelenburg. The eyes, while seen in the mirrors of the prone view, were not protected. The head should have been taken off the prone view every 30 min. Ischemic neuropathy is the most common cause of vision loss. Ischemic optic neuropathy may present as anterior (involving ischemia and infarction of the intraocular optic nerve) or posterior (involving ischemia and infarction of the intraorbital optic nerve). Increased and sustained intraocular pressure causes ischemia. Blindness is usually irreversible.

Robert was probably blind in one eye from central artery occlusion. It is usually caused by pressure improperly related to pressure on the eye from positioning. Pressure on the eye increases IOP and decreases blood flow to the retina through the central retinal artery. The increased IOP exceeds the perfusion pressure of the central retinal artery, leading to ischemia of the retina. Most patients with central retinal artery occlusion develop a unilateral, permanent blindness.

Many risk factors for postoperative vision loss have been identified that include older patients, elevated baseline IOPs, hypertension, diabetes, obesity, anemia, vascular disease, increased blood viscosity, smokers, intraoperative hypotension, blood transfusions, lower colloid use during fluid administration, and prolonged surgical times.

Robert was positioned on a horseshoe-shaped headrest prone pillow. The head should be slightly in extension, and there was a mirror at the base to visualize the patient's eyes and the mouth. Patients who are predisposed to acute angle-closure glaucoma are also at high risk for ocular injury even during short procedures. The prone position can shift the lens-iris diaphragm forward so it obstructs aqueous humor outflow and increases IOP. Most cases of blindness after surgery occur in the geriatric population.

Mike Moss asked an interesting question. "Should patients designated for the prone position have their intraocular pressures checked prior to surgery." While there is no data on this subject, it seemed more than reasonable. There is no resource utilization issue as the number of patients per day, at most, would be 2–3 patients having the IOPs checked a day in the presurgical testing.

Robert had resilience. He would adapt and live with one eye. His back was painful, but he worked through it. Jalen had connections with Tulane and Trinity. The complexities of his courses increased, as well as his GPA. Robert's cumulative GPA was 3.45, and the essay on his application was inspirational. He was able to move forward with a case of intraoperative blindness. Robert was accepted to the Trinity School of Medicine without Jalen's connection.

This was a rare but preventable severe complication. He never felt handicapped but was extremely on edge when a new "glass eye" replaced his injured eye. He looked "cross-eyed" for the rest of his life.

Suggested Reading

1. Chandra KN, et al. Visual loss after cervical laminectomy in the prone position. Rev Bras Anestesiol. 2017;67(4):435–8. PMID: 28433204 Portuguese.
2. Epstein NE. How to avoid perioperative visual loss following prone spinal surgery. Surg Neurol Int. 2016;7(Suppl 13):S328–30. https://doi.org/10.4103/2152-7806.182543. eCollection 2016. PMID: 27274406.

3. Kwee MM, Ho YH, Rozen WM. The prone position during surgery and its complications: a systematic review and evidence-based guidelines. Int Surg. 2015;100(2):292–303. https://doi.org/10.9738/INTSURG-D-13-00256.1. PMID: 25692433.
4. Ooi EIL, et al. Unilateral visual loss after spine surgery in the prone position for extradural haematoma in a healthy young man. BMJ Case Rep. 2013;2013:bcr2013200632. PMID: 24334521.

32 Anesthesia and a Grand Mal Seizure and Intracranial Hypotension

Cary Musgrave

Cary clunked her way into the room, and all of the guests at the table stood and gave Cary the standing ovation that she deserved. She was still winning her battle that started at birth. Apparently, something went wrong in the delivery room, and Cary was deprived of oxygen somewhere in the birth canal. Her APGAR score was 4/7, and she was intubated and on a ventilator for a month. While she was full term, the prolonged (nobody knows how long) period of anoxia left her body wounded for the rest of her life.

Her diagnosis was cerebral palsy. Her gait and hand control were devastated. One leg was shorter, and her hands were spastic. As long as she could walk, the sole of one shoe was adjusted to add inches to match her other leg. The lengthened leg always clunked when she walked. She mastered walking with multiple adjustments to defy gravity.

Cary's left hand hosted fingers were bent and stiff. The dexterity was just not there. Her speech was a bit garbled, but it was only noticeable by those who knew her.

Cary Musgrave grew up in the black neighborhood of Jackson, Mississippi. Cerebral palsy skipped her brain. She was simply brilliant. Her razor-sharp mind always distracted those who were just getting to know her. Her parents sold fresh fruits and vegetables out of a stand. It was a hard go, living on the poor side of Jackson, but their work ethic transformed their vegetable stand to become the provider of stunning vegetables and fruit to many of the "famous" restaurants in Mississippi and Louisiana. The Brennan empire of restaurants in New Orleans relied on their ingredients from the 1980s until today. Cary grew up working the stand until college and spent all of her summers working with her parents.

Children can be more than mean, and Cary was teased, threatened, and the center of too many biting jokes. She blossomed in her adolescence and became a beautiful young woman.

Cary had the choice of any university. She compensated for her physical disability and used her mind to equal the playing field. Her parents encouraged her to aim

C. Scher, *Anesthesia Conversations*,
https://doi.org/10.1007/978-3-032-05354-1_32

high and not feel any intimidation in her life. Cassie chose Vanderbilt and majored in physics.

There were two events that changed her life and her self-image, giving her a level of confidence that would never leave her tortured body. Cary made the women's track team. She ran the 100-meter sprint and always came in last. Her coach was unwavering and made sure that she was in every race.

The team rallied around her after every loss. She cried out of sheer happiness. She also found a remarkably dedicated physical therapist who worked at her college, and with twice-daily strengthening and mobility sessions. Her arm and hand dexterity was at the level of most of her classmates.

In her third year, a member of the men's track team asked her out on a date. A real date. Earl Washington was from Alexandria, Louisiana, and saw a beautiful woman in Cary. He was a political science major and had a vision of being in the House of Representatives in a district that was 100%. African American in an impoverished area in Orleans Parish. His political dream became a reality only 5 years after graduation. Earl Washington married Cary, who became Cary Washington.

Cary's vision of her life was to better the lives of those who had handicaps. She met the Dean of Student Affairs at Tulane University School of Medicine. After a 30-minute discussion, she was accepted to the medical school with a full scholarship. Cary acknowledged but refused the scholarship. Her parents had become wealthy, and Cary wanted her 4-year "free ride" to be offered to another student who was in need. She was grateful for Tulane's prestigious reputation and for Earl who was in their law school.

Lily was smitten with Cary and made sure that she could match for her anesthesia residency and neuroanesthesia fellowship. Cary rose to become the Director of Neuroanesthesia at Trinity. Her three consecutive teacher of the year awards were a testament to her commitment to teaching residents and medical students.

Cary was a bit annoyed when the operating room schedule came out. While she was the Director of Neuroanesthesia, she was assigned to the inguinal hernia room. There were three consecutive hernias, and the surgeon did not want a spinal, epidural, or simple local injections into the surgical field. In the last year, he had four cases of urinary retention from a spinal, three wet taps from an epidural (all required a blood patch), and one case where intralipid was administered for local anesthetic systemic toxicity.

"Just put them to sleep" was the opening remark by Jim Baine, the Chair of General Surgery. He was dismissive of every anesthesiologist. He thought that general anesthesia was fine for most of his patients unless the anesthesia team had a specific and reasonable concern. Cary thought the case was not ideal for a senior resident and was assigned to be the solo attending in the room along with a medical student. Working with medical students was ideal, as Cary always enjoyed the enthusiasm of the students, whether they chose anesthesia or some other field of medicine.

For the third case, a 58-year-old man presented for an open repair of an inguinal hernia. The surgeon believed that his open repairs were better than his laparoscopic repairs. The patient reported no significant medical problems, including allergies. He was on no medications. He did not remember when he last went for an annual medical checkup. His presurgical Covid test was negative. He was not accompanied by a family member or a family friend.

The patient reported to the surgery center and had complied with the NPO policy. The electronic anesthesia record from his clinical record was empty. Cary came by and introduced herself. She did a brief physical exam, including an airway evaluation that was unremarkable. On the patient's bed was a paper towel from the bathroom in the preoperative holding area. The first blood pressure was written down on the paper towel by the holding area nurse was 230/110. The handwriting of the vital signs was poor. Cary read them as 130/110. There was no communication between the nurse who wrote the vitals on the paper and Cary. The blood pressure was repeated and again was 230/110. Cary chose to proceed. Anesthesia plus an antihypertensive would solve the problem. Two milligrams of Midazolam lowered the blood pressure to 160/90.

"Were these the vitals taken on our patient? The first blood pressure in the operating room was 210/100." Cary's medical student arrived at the bedside and was shocked by the blood pressure. Cary administered another 2 mg midazolam and waited 10 min for the midazolam to kick in. The next blood pressure was 170/100.

Cary and her medical student agreed that anxiety was driving his blood pressure up. This was probably close to the patient's baseline blood pressure; medical management and optimization could take months. Although the case was not urgent, the patient did need the surgery to avoid the risk of later bowel incarceration.

For any patient who did not have a primary care physician, the surgery was rarely canceled on the day of surgery. There was always the risk, in an underserved hospital, of the patient not showing up for surgery again. Being an NPO, overcoming anxiety to come to the hospital, language and cultural barriers were often deterrents for a smooth and safe clinical experience. Men and women of color are more likely to refuse neuraxial anesthesia compared with their white counterparts. The patient was relieved that the anesthesiologist did not sell the epidural.

The duration of the case was an hour. The anesthetic started with 100 mg of esmolol to blunt the hemodynamic response to intubation. The pressure changed minimally, but the pulse decreased to 67 beats per minute. A routine anesthetic was administered: cefazolin, lidocaine, propofol, hydromorphone, rocuronium, sevoflurane, dexamethasone, ondansetron, and sugammadex. The vitals during the case were systolic between 130 and 140 and a pulse of 68. At extubation, the final blood pressure in the operating room was 140/90.

Cary thought that her willingness to proceed was the right thing to do.

The initial blood pressure in the PACU was 156/90. Three minutes later, the blood pressure was 186/90. The assumption by the PACU resident and attending was that the patient was in pain.

Increments of 0.2 mg of hydromorphone were administered. The blood pressure rose to 212/95 mmHg. The assumption again was that pain was the culprit. Small doses of hydromorphone were titrated to effect. The patient was alert, comfortable, and yet still extremely hypertensive.

Everyone involved in the care of the patient was now in shock. The patient had a massive Grand Mal Seizure. The PACU resident gave 200 mg of propofol, and the seizure was terminated. The blood pressure in the postictal state was 290/100. A nicardipine drip was started, and the patient was sent for a CT-angio scan that revealed a subarachnoid hemorrhage with blood that emanated from the posterior communicating artery.

The patient was transported to the Neurosurgical Intensive Care Unit. An external ventricular drain (EVD) was placed, and cerebral spinal fluid (CSF) would be drawn off if the CSF pressure was above 20 mmHg. The CSF pressure was 27 mm/Hg, and 50 cc was drawn off every 10 min for a total of 100 cc. The neurology team did a comprehensive examination and discovered bilateral "blown pupils" that were unresponsive to light and absent corneal reflexes. The exam is an assessment of sensorium, cognition, cranial nerves, motor, sensory, cerebellar reflexes, and meningeal irritation. Cary did her own Glasgow Coma Scale exam, which evaluates eye opening, best motor response, and best sensory response. The patient's Glasgow was below 8.

The patient did not fit the criteria of 'brain dead" but was severely compromised. The neurosurgical chief said, if you are going to have an aneurysm burst, the posterior communicating artery causes a lesser neurologic impairment. While it was early after the rupture, the neurosurgeons were optimistic.

Cary was devastated that she allowed this case to move forward despite the initial vital signs. Blood pressure management caused the aneurysm to burst. All people have aneurysms, but they must be greater than 5 cm to be at risk of bursting. This explanation did not change Cary's self-inflicted guilt.

The following day, at 6:00 in the morning, Cary came to the unit to see the patient.

"Holy shit!! He is tracking. Wherever my face moves, his eyes follow." She was ecstatic. While intubated, he was trying to talk. Cary extubated the patient, and he responded. His initial sentences made no sense, but each day he would grasp for words and put a coherent sentence together. By day seven, he was discharged and had an appointment with speech therapy.

The members of the root cause analysis (RCA) service met and found that there was no breach of care. Most voted that they would have done the same. His initial blood sugar was 200. His LFTs were elevated in preop testing. His PSA was 0.7.

Cary was given a time bomb. Despite the judgment of the RCA, she felt enormous guilt. She could have switched the order of the patients, which would have allowed for blood pressure evaluation and treatment. The ball was dropped when she did not look for the patient's true blood pressure on the paper towel. She blamed herself and not the nurse.

Prior to discharge, an appointment was made for the patient to be fully evaluated in the medicine clinic. An EKG, echocardiography, metabolic panel, PSA, CBC, and B12 were ordered. The nurse who wrote vital signs on a paper towel without mentioning it to Cary was reprimanded.

Suggested Reading

1. Gil-Garcia CA, Flores-Alvarez E, Cebrian-Garcia R, Mendoza-Lopez AC, Gonzalez-Hermosillo LM, Garcia-Blanco MD, Roldan-Valadez E. Essential topics about imaging diagnosis and treatment of hemorrhagic stroke: a comprehensive review of the 2022 guidelines. Curr Probl Cardiol. 2022;47(11):101328. https://doi.org/10.1016/j.cpcar.
2. Hanada S, Kawakami H, Goto T, Morita S. Hypertension and anesthesia. Curr Opin Anaesthesiol. 2006;19(3):315–9. https://doi.org/10.1097/01.aco.0000192811.56161.23.
3. Inagawa T. Prevalence of cerebral aneurysms in autopsy studies: a review of the literature. Neurosurg Rev. 2022;45(4):2565–82. https://doi.org/10.1007/s10143-022-01783-7. Epub 2022 Apr 22.
4. Marcucci M, Chan MTV, Smith EE, Absalom AR, Devereaux PJ. Prevention of perioperative stroke in patients undergoing non-cardiac surgery. Lancet Neurol. 2023;22(10):946–58. https://doi.org/10.1016/S1474-4422(23)00209-0. PMID: 37739575 Review.
5. Spence JD. Controlling resistant hypertension. Stroke Vasc Neurol. 2018;3(2):69–75. https://doi.org/10.1136/svn-2017-000138. eCollection 2018 Jun.

Biomedical Research and Iris's Stroke Recovery

33

Iris Goldsmith

Iris was the model resident in her class. In her final year of cardiac anesthesia fellowship, her next-door neighbor called the department of anesthesia at 11 PM and stated that Iris was sick and would be out for the next day. At the age of 31, Iris had a stroke. Iris was found on the floor of her bathroom around 6 PM by her neighbor who dropped by to pay Iris back for the 100 dollars that she owed. The front door of the apartment was usually unlocked, and the shower was running with steaming hot water. Iris was aphasic and could not move the dominant right side of her body. There were tears, and from the look on her face, the tears were not new. Her skin became scalded. She could not move her legs. It was not possible to determine when the stroke began.

An ambulance from Trinity Hospital had three providers. A neck collar was placed, and the oxygen flow rate was set at 8 liters in a non-rebreathing mask. An intravenous was placed. The hospital was notified that the stroke team should be in the emergency department to receive her.

A neurological exam was followed by a CT angiogram. The diagnosis was a subarachnoid bleed from the left frontal-temporal part of the brain. There was a modest displacement of the lateral ventricles of the brain, implying that there was intracranial hypertension. An EVD (external ventricular drain) was inserted to both measure intracranial pressure and to draw off CSF if the pressure was excessive. There was evidence of vasospasm at the site of the bleed, and the neuro-interventional radiology (NIR) team planned a cerebral angiogram with intravascular injections of nimodipine in areas of vasospasm.

A general anesthetic was planned. The anesthesia team inserted a preinduction arterial line, and 1 mg/kg of esmolol was administered to block the hemodynamic discharge for intubation. The pulse started at 87 and within 2 min, dropped to 76. Every patient has a different fully beta-blocked pulse. The anesthesiology team was ready to induce, believing that 76 was her fully beta-blocked pulse.

There were some hemodynamic changes, and the systemic blood pressure increased from 150/90 to 160/94. A nicardipine infusion was set up to control her

C. Scher, *Anesthesia Conversations*,
https://doi.org/10.1007/978-3-032-05354-1_33

pressure. With fluoroscopy, there was no change in the initial images after the intubation.

With IV contrast, there was mild bleeding at the site of an aneurysm. Her entire cerebral circulation was littered with small aneurysms. The neuroradiologist said that everyone has aneurysms. The size of those aneurysms makes them inconsequential, and life goes on. Iris's aneurysm was greater than 5 cm, and with an increase in blood pressure, there theoretically was a chance of rupture. The aerobic exercise that she did in the morning probably increased her blood pressure and "burst" the walls of this particular aneurysm.

After three days, her aphasia improved. Iris was "reaching" for words. She would compose a logical sentence, but there were frequent words that had nothing to do with reality. Rather than saying that "I will walk the dog," she said "I will walk the door." Her right leg was judged to be a second-degree burn that was improving slowly each day. She struggled with her right arm, particularly with her hand. It just "hung" as if it were not part of her body.

After weeks of hard-core rehab, the hand appeared to be a lost cause. Iris was told by several colleagues at work that her days of practicing anesthesia were over. Anesthesia is heavy on procedures that need both hands. She considered an amputation of her hand and replacement with a somewhat functional prosthesis. Her rehabilitation team suggested that amputation would be a last resort. Iris needed a second opinion.

Dr. Max Shapiro was the Director of Stroke Rehabilitation at the Fischer Institute in Rochester, Minnesota. For the last 10 years, he has served on the FDA Committee for Biomedical Research. He leads a research team that determines the efficacy of biomedical products to aid stroke patients before they are released to the public. His clinical focus is on devices that will improve the recovery of stroke victims. Chris did legwork necessary to get an appointment for Iris with Dr. Shapiro.

Dr. Shapiro did a comprehensive history and physical on Iris. He reviewed her previous therapy. "Iris, I need to know your goals for your recovery. You have a foot drop and several hand issues. I think with some of the new biomedical devices, you will be able to pursue your career in anesthesiology. We should be able to see the efficacy of these new devices in less than a month. None of these devices are unsafe. I also have products in trials and we can look at those. There is no cost for these devices and I will not charge you for my services. Although all have been cleared by the FDA, I need to see them work in scores of patents.

We will start with the 'Neural Sleeve' for your foot drop (Cionic company). The mechanism is electrostimulation. Let me read the information on their website; precisely coordinated to the gait cycle and software-steered."

Functional stimulation is delivered to the four major muscle groups of the leg: hamstring, quadriceps, calf, and shin. The system knows when you're sitting, standing, or walking, providing the right stimulation at the right time. The system continuously optimizes stimulation patterns to make each step smarter than the last. Let's call CIONIC now for an appointment. My guess is that they will work with you in less than a week.

Now onto your arm. There is a company called VIVISTIM that has a product for vagus nerve stimulation in strokes. It works by sending electrical impulses through the vagus nerve, which triggers a cascade in the brain, primarily promoting neuroplasticity, meeting the brain's ability to reorganize and form new neural connections. The goal is to improve motor functions in areas of the stroke for the upper limbs. Physical therapy releases neurotransmitters like acetylcholine and norepinephrine that have anti-inflammatory and neuroprotective properties. The combination of PT and vagus nerve stimulation works synergistically for optimal recovery.

"The company that makes this device is Vivistim. I will contact them today. I will also get you a pair of robotic gloves.

Robotic gloves are suitable for the patients with hand dysfunction such as stroke, hemiplegia after cerebral infarction, peripheral nerve injury of hand, orthopedic surgery, spinal cord injury hand burn, children cerebral palsy, etc. There is now an explosion of technical science that is more natural than gloves but is still in the testing stage.

Robotic gloves combine flexible robot technology and neuroscience. It helps with finger flexion and extension, reduces hand muscle tension, relieves edema and stiffness, promotes rehabilitation of brain nerve injury through exercise, and improves hand activity and accelerate the rehabilitation of hand function. The cost of a glove is approximately 300 dollars."

It took two exhausting years of physical therapy and modern technology to give her the confidence to have a career in Chris's department. Iris could intubate, practice neuraxial anesthesia, read TEEs, and set up an operating room for any case. She was a self-proclaimed expert at regional anesthesia. Central lines were not an issue, but peripheral IVs were a challenge. Trinity has a great academic program with a full complement of residents who could do whatever she could not. At the two-year mark, she felt as "normal" as she was going to get. She would find her place in anesthesia.

Iris contacted Chris for a position during her fellowship year. Chris met with her before the stroke and a month later, after her stroke. He did not think she would be able to take on the physical rigors of practicing anesthesia. He checked in with her periodically and was inspired by her drive to return to work. Iris took Chris out to lunch every 6 months after her stroke. Chris was amazed by the ongoing improvement from the biomedical devices and Iris's power-packed drive to become part again, at Trinity Anesthesia.

Iris wanted to open up a clinic for physically impaired physicians. It was not a pipedream. She partnered up with both Trinity and Tulane to have a dedicated area in Tulane Hospital for the center. Iris had an exhaustive list of necessary items. Having the highest qualified staff was essential, and that would be expensive.

From inception, the center opened two years later. All on-site treatments were of no cost. The only requirement was to bring to the center documentation of the injury and treatments that were previously attempted. The center was funded by private donations, the State of Louisiana and the US government. Iris practiced anesthesia three times a week, and two days were dedicated to the clinic and fundraising. She felt peace of mind that her near-tragic stroke helped so many of her fellow physicians.

Suggested Reading

1. Fesk K. Ischemic stroke. Am J Med. 2021;134(12):1457–64. https://doi.org/10.1016/j.amjmed.2021.07.027. Epub 2021 Aug 27.
2. Klamroth-Marganska V. Stroke rehabilitation: therapy robots and assisted devices. Adv Exp Med Biol. 2018;1065:579–87. https://doi.org/10.1007/978-3-319-77932-4_35. PMID: 30051408 Review.
3. Ko MJ, Chuang YC, Ou-Yang LJ, Cheng YY, Tsai YL, Lee YC. The application of soft robotic gloves in stroke patients: a systematic review and meta-analysis of randomized controlled trials. Brain Sci. 2023;13(6):900. https://doi.org/10.3390/brainsci13060900. PMID: 37371378.
4. Malakouti N, Serruya MD, Cramer SC, Kimberley TJ, Rosenwasser RH. Making sense of vagus nerve stimulation for stroke. Stroke. 2024;55(2):519–22. https://doi.org/10.1161/STROKEAHA.123.044576. Epub 20.
5. Proulx CE, Higgins J, Vincent C, Vaughan T, Hewko M, Gagnon DH. User-centered development process of an operating interface to couple a robotic glove with virtual environment to optimize hand rehabilitation following a stroke. J Rehabil Assist Technol Eng. 2023;10:20556683231166574. https://doi.org/10.1177/20556683231166574. eCollection 2023 Jan–Dec.
6. Rodríguez-Fernández A, Lobo-Prat J, Font-Llagunes JM. Systematic review on wearable lower-limb exoskeletons for gait training in neuromuscular impairments. J Neuroeng Rehabil. 2021;18(1):22. https://doi.org/10.1186/s12984-021-00815-5. PMID: 33526065.
7. Winstein CJ, Stein J, Arena R, Bates B, Cherney LR, Cramer SC, Deruyter F, Eng JJ, Fisher B, Harvey RL, Lang CE, MacKay-Lyons M, Ottenbacher KJ, Pugh S, Reeves MJ, Richards LG, Stiers W, Zorowitz RD; American Heart Association Stroke Council, Council on Cardiovascular and Stroke Nursing, Council on Clinical Cardiology, and Council on Quality of Care and Outcomes Research. Guidelines for adult stroke rehabilitation and recovery: a guideline for healthcare professionals from the American Heart Association/American Stroke Association. Stroke. 2016;47(6):e98–e169. https://doi.org/10.1161/STR.0000000000000098.

Anesthesia and Sensorial Hearing Loss 34

Seth Grant

Seth Grant was awarded to the State of Louisiana when it was determined that both parents were unable to function as parents as a result of their own substance abuse and not providing an atmosphere that was safe for their 3-year-old son. There were no medical records, including a vaccination schedule. Seth was in the tenth percentile for height and weight. He looked malnourished to anyone who took a minute to look at him.

The Chief of Pediatrics at Ochsner determined that it was likely that Seth never received vaccinations. Serology determined that the antibodies of the measles vaccine are much lower than those of a measles infection. Serology was determined for each childhood disease. There were no antibodies for mumps, rubella, diphtheria, Haemophilus influenzae type b, and pertussis. By serology, he had the measles that caused severe auditory nerve damage. He was deaf for the rest of his life. Hearing aids and cochlear implants require a functioning auditory nerve. There were no devices to help Seth's handicap.

The Grants were truly a gift from above. They took on the role that could challenge them for the rest of their lives, but they did not see it that way. They hung on tight to their gift.

Like so many deaf people, Seth could not moderate his speech. His speech therapist improved his pitch and tone, but Seth did not have the confidence to speak. The Grants spent a fortune providing every device and professional to make Seth have a great and big life.

Seth and the Grants connected from day one. Goal number one was to get Seth healthy: vaccinations, nourishment, socialization, inclusion, and acceptance. At the age of four, Seth entered mainstream education for the deaf. He found his new best friend, an 8-week-old Golden Retriever puppy. Seth's mother found the puppy more of a challenge than Seth.

Seth excelled in every grade in school. He was an excellent athlete and played every sport with hearing children. His father tipped the scales toward golf and tennis—two sports where the hearing had no advantage over the non-hearing. His

C. Scher, *Anesthesia Conversations*,
https://doi.org/10.1007/978-3-032-05354-1_34

mother was an accomplished artist, favoring ceramics, sculpture, painting, and photography. Seth was immersed in all of these endeavors.

Caroline was the name of his first and forever girlfriend. They became inseparable in high school and chose to attend the University of Michigan together with its superior curriculum for the deaf. They both shared the vision that scholastic achievement would elevate them above the hearing students, and they were correct. They both were accepted to Brown School of Medicine with 100% support by their classmates. All lectures were online with subtitles, and clinical rotations were done together with the help of a sign expert.

Seth and Caroline's families, professors, and friends thought that they should strongly consider a field of medicine that was easiest on their handicap: radiology, pathology, and possibly dermatology. Seth chose anesthesiology, and Caroline chose Public Health. In both choices, they made life even more complicated.

Seth's plan would be to hire a person with perfect sign skills to help Seth respond to the challenges needed when a critical crisis occurs in the operating room. The "sign" person had to be familiar with the language of medicine specific to anesthesia.

Seth was used to his turbulent life hurdles. What program in the National Residency Matching Program would be willing to be burdened with a deaf student who needs rapid critical responses to communicate with surgeons, nurses, consultants, and families?

Seth's USMLE scores were superior compared to most of his medical classmates, but his clinical rotations suffered. He was, compared to his classmates, as "just passing" for the most important rotations in medical school. He had a wide array of coping mechanisms, but they did not match the needs of clinical duty. After 6 months of suffering, his family hired a sign person who did some sign language for both a surgeon and an internist. His anesthesia rotation was the least problematic for the patients and for his colleagues. His sign person, Robert, had some experience with medicine and he was able to keep up the pace of the busy operating room.

Due to his handicap, he applied to 60 anesthesia programs. Anesthesiology was the most challenging for his handicap, but he had a plan.

Seth had six invitations in Anesthesiology: Trinity, Mount Sinai, MGH, Johns Hopkins, Yale, and Brown. These programs were willing to take a gamble. The Yale interview was the first. Robert, a sign language expert, rode with Seth on the 90-minute Amtrak ride from Grand Central Station and practiced a wide range of interview questions that could come up. Out of anxiety, Seth was signing at a pace that Robert could not keep up. Robert insisted that Seth slow it down and practice with a metronome. While Seth could not hear the metronome, he followed the pendulum bar. Robert adjusted the bar at a pace where Seth looked relaxed. Seth, with Robert, had to answer appropriate but difficult questions at his interview. They were both nervous.

Yale was willing to help Seth in any way possible. Seth's nerves got the best of him, and he became frightened. Yale wanted Seth, but he was clearly spooked. He called Yale and thanked them for an excellent day and their willingness to take a gamble on his handicap. Seth withdrew his application. Seth did not want so much attention during his residency. He realized that one mistake could be catastrophic. He questioned his choice of Anesthesiology. He cancelled all of his interviews.

Seth's parents thought he had done the right thing by cancelling. He decided to look at pathology programs. He could easily function without professional liability in that field. If he needed an interpreter, that would be easy.

There was a cocktail party for all of the Chairs of Anesthesia in the USA at the Annual Meeting of the American Society of Anesthesia in San Francisco. Chris was a "Master of the Universe" at cocktail parties. He was an all-star "mingler" and could join any group of people seamlessly. Chris naturally joined a group, and Seth was the topic of conversation. Lily told Chris that Seth cancelled his interview. Three Chairs in the group were in agreement that there were many upsides of having Seth on their service. There were several possible downsides. Concern for patient care was the bottom line. "To be perfectly clear, why even go there!"

Chris stepped away and texted Lily. "Find Seth! We have his application. Give me his cell number. We need to talk to him and his family."

Lily responded within minutes. Chris made the call. Chris rehearsed what he wanted to say over and over. This was a conversation that had to be clear, unwavering, and relaxed.

"Can I have a chance to meet Seth? I want you both to come to New Orleans with Seth. I would not have made this call unless I was sure that we could provide him an atmosphere where he will feel comfortable training, make everlasting friendships, engage in academic activities, and guarantee his marketability. He will have the opportunity to join the faculty if he chooses that path."

Seth's parents were speechless.

"My team will contact you for times when you are free to come to New Orleans. Everything will be arranged from flights to hotels, to meals, to local transportation and whatever else I can think of.

You will be staying at the Four Seasons and you will need a jacket and tie for one dinner."

"We would like to come next week. Is that too early? Can we bring Caroline, his girlfriend for life?"

"Of course. Perfect!"

It had to be Commander's. Chris made the reservation and remembered to order the Bread Pudding when he arrived at the restaurant. He stuck to his rule of getting to the restaurant early to grab a drink signaling that it was fine to calm the nerves with a scotch or two if need be. Chris let it be known that it was fine to order alcohol at most of life's events. He held his own and had a drink or two before a funeral.

"I heard your story, and I cannot find a single reason for you not to train with us. To be clear, our department will have no obstacles in your training. You will be a resident and the department will pay for anything you need to make you whole. If you need someone to sign for you, we will find several people who can sign. You will never be without someone who can sign. Over time, your facial appearance and body language will be a significant way of communication. Sign language will be a requirement for our residents.

Caroline, I believe we have the resources to pursue any career path you choose. Our Public Health Department has an international reputation for excellence. Of course you will have a position there if you choose to do so. While Seth will be meeting a "bunch" of people tomorrow, we can arrange a fruitful visit for you with the leadership of our Public Health Department."

After 4 years of residency and a year of a regional fellowship, Seth joined the faculty and learned every day how to make it easier for a seamless conversation and communication. He would be a Trinity lifer.

Chris' reputation for training those who have a physical handicap made his already national reputation soar. There are always openings for Chair positions in the country at some of the most prestigious medical schools that offered him interviews. He always declined. He, like most from New Orleans, never left New Orleans. He had created a special niche for residents with physical handicaps.

Suggested Reading

1. Agaronnik N, Campbell EG, Ressalam J, Iezzoni LI. Communicating with patients with disability: perspectives of practicing physicians. J Gen Intern Med. 2019;34(7):1139–45. https://doi.org/10.1007/s11606-019-04911-0. Epub 2019 Mar 18. PMID: 30887435.
2. McGlade K, et al. Deaf awareness training in medical schools. Med Teach. 2013;35(9):789–90. PMID: 23968320.
3. McKee MM, Smith S, Barnett S, et al. What are the benefits of training deaf and hard of hearing doctors? Acad Med. 2013;88(2):158–61. https://doi.org/10.1097/ACM.0b013e31827c0aef. PMID: 23361028.
4. Paatsch L, Toe D. The Impact of pragmatic delays for deaf and hard of hearing students in mainstream classrooms. Pediatrics. 2020;146(Suppl 3):S292–7. https://doi.org/10.1542/peds.2020-0242I. PMID: 33139443.
5. Saidia AR, Ruel J, Bahloul A, Chaix B, Venail F, Wang J. Current advances in gene therapies of genetic auditory neuropathy spectrum disorder. J Clin Med. 2023;12(3):738. https://doi.org/10.3390/jcm12030738. PMID: 36769387.

Fraud

35

Jack Stone

Tara and Olive were put off by him during his Trinity residency. The more Jack Stone talked, the weirder he sounded. During his time at Trinity, he did not show an interest in anesthesiology which was transparent from his lack of any communication skills. Jack functioned at a high level, but his long moments of silence damaged his credibility. His fellowship in pain management and three years as an attending at Vanderbilt were productive yet made him homesick for his life back in New Orleans. He wanted to return to Trinity. Chris thought that Jack was brilliant, but within minutes of being with him alone, he seemed to have a "screw loose."

Lily would have rather waited for another faculty applicant who was not bizarre. Chris needed more attendings to get the residency off probation. Jack always showed potential as a resident, and Chris believed that with mentoring, his potential would be unleashed. In time, Chris found out that Jack could not be mentored. When Jack's story came out, he was terminated.

Steven Craft, the editor in chief of the journal "Anesthesia and Analgesia," noticed that there were frequent papers, or better stated, too many research papers over a short period by Jack Stone. Steve looked up Jack on PUBMED. The papers were always about different strategies for postoperative and chronic pain management. Jack was the first author of each paper, and a man with the same last name was the second author. He was Jack's father. There was never a third author.

Steve Craft reviewed each paper. They were all algorithms or better stated, recipes, if followed, would eliminate the need for postoperative narcotics. There are new regulations that some state medical boards mandate that narcotics must be electronically prescribed, for only five days with documentation for more days if needed. Prescribers were being "tracked" at a time the opioid crisis ran out of control. Jack's papers made it easier to follow the regulations and at the same time, delivered a patient-centered approach. Steve reviewed 13 papers by Stone. They were perfectly written with seamless statistics. The conclusions and summaries were too good to be true. The science in the papers was referenced, and all followed sequentially.

C. Scher, *Anesthesia Conversations*,
https://doi.org/10.1007/978-3-032-05354-1_35

Craft was concerned that if the algorithms were followed, patient care would change around the world, for the worse.

Steve called for a meeting for the editorial board to investigate Jack's published works. His staff made a PowerPoint presentation that aimed to bring out the facts. While Jack was innocent until proven guilty, an oversight legal team was there to make sure that all of the rules of an investigation were enforced. There were six slides for each paper. Each paper was too good to be true. The committee was sure that the entire content of the papers was "made up." The pattern of each clinical question, hypotheses, experimental design, data analysis, and manuscript preparation were all just too similar.

Each paper had a similar formula. They each gave a recipe for postoperative pain management. Legal reported that the presentation was worthy of a path that leads to the next step in the investigation, onto the formation of a Grand Jury and an oversight legal team to ensure the rules of the Grand Jury were obeyed. The Grand Jury came to the conclusion that Jack should be indicted within 15 min after Jack's case was presented. A court date was set.

Jack's trial lasted three days in court, which did not bode well for him. The judge concluded that: 1. The papers were entirely fictional and were 100% supported by Big Pharma. 2. The second author was Jack's father who was a Professor of Clinical Trials and Translational Medicine at an Ivy League medical school. He was the expert on the selection of a particular experimental design that matches the goals of each "made-up" treatment. 3. Physicians who read these manuscripts are using the false data to treat their own patients. 4. There were no more than 10 citations per paper. Chris deleted his application for a Trinity position.

Jack ultimately pled guilty to fraud with numerous counts of violations. His fictitious data inflicted pain on patients who were receiving care from physicians whose practice was based on hundreds of lies. There was no path for a plea.

Jack was sentenced to a low-security prison for 18 months and was fined 100,000 dollars. Neither component had any real impact on his financial status. He had received millions of dollars for many years from drug companies and device manufacturers. Jack's license to practice medicine was rescinded in Massachusetts, Pennsylvania, and Louisiana. Why did it take so long to see the pattern? All 50 states were notified in a short secure email to refute the findings in the papers. Each governor's office decided how to deliver the facts to the general public.

All of the states joined in by denying any attempt from Jack of getting a license in their state. Jack's days of practicing medicine were over. When asked about not being a doctor again, he gave the response: "I don't give a shit."

Anesthesiologists are not psychiatrists, but over the years, it was clear that Jack had some sort of mood disorder. There was a consensus among the nurses and doctors that at baseline, he was always a "bit depressed" and a loner. He was kind to his patients but empathy seemed to be missing. He was just off the bell-shaped curve, or better stated, he was "next to normal." None of his coresidents at Trinity disliked him nor liked him. He was more than under the radar, and the residents respected him.

Prison was not kind to Jack. The tremor that he had for years worsened. He was later diagnosed with Parkinson's Disease. He never returned to medicine again.

Parkinson's is a progressive disorder that is caused by degeneration of nerve cells in the part of the brain called the substantia nigra, which controls movement. These nerve cells lose the ability to produce dopamine. Studies have shown that symptoms of Parkinson's develop in patients with an 80% or greater loss of dopamine-producing cells in the substantia nigra.

Dopamine operates in balance with other neurotransmitters to coordinate the millions of nerve and muscle cells involved in movement. Without enough dopamine, this balance is disrupted, resulting in tremor, rigidity, slowness of movement, impaired balance, and coordination.

Jack never felt remorse for his crimes. He believed that over time, his fraudulent papers would be forgotten. When asked later in his life about his version of his actions, he always replied that he was forced to act by Big Pharma.

In the last year of his life, he went to an emergency room for acute appendicitis. He was aware of his autonomic dysfunction; The anesthesiologist had to consider orthostatic hypotension, sialorrhea, incontinence, and excessive sweating. Autonomic instability can lead to sudden, exaggerated, or uncertain responses to central neuraxial blockade.

Respiratory dysfunction results from the uncoordinated involuntary movement as a result of rigidity and muscle weakness. Pharyngeal muscle weakness leads to increased retention and impaired expulsion of respiratory secretions that can cause perioperative aspiration pneumonia.

Jack's gastrointestinal symptoms included medication-induced nausea and gastroesophageal reflux. Preoperative acid aspiration prophylaxis is desired with a rapid sequence induction in those patients with advanced disease.

Neuropsychiatric symptoms include changes in mood, cognition, and behavior. Psychotic symptoms include delusions and hallucinations. These symptoms can lead to postoperative emergence reactions, and with associated tremors and rigidity, can lead to dilemmas at the time of extubation. Most of the exacerbations related to an anesthetic occur and more advanced stages than his. He moved forward with a laparoscopic appendectomy. Two attending physicians operated, and there was no impact on the surgery or Jack's state of Parkinson's.

Two years after the appendectomy, he was put in hospice and passed away only weeks later. He was correct in saying that all of his transgressions would be forgotten within 5 years. He was incorrect.

Suggested Reading

1. Costa HN, Esteves AR, Empadinhas N, Cardoso SM. Parkinson's disease: a multisystem disorder. Neurosci Bull. 2023;39(1):113–24. https://doi.org/10.1007/s12264-022-00934-6. Epub 2022 Aug 22. PMID: 35994167 Review.
2. Katzenschlager R, Hallett M, Poewe W. Pharmacological treatment of tremor in Parkinson's disease revisited. J Parkinsons Dis. 2023;13(2):127–44. https://doi.org/10.3233/JPD-225060.
3. Meng D, Jin Z, Wang Y, Fang B. Longitudinal cognitive changes in patients with early Parkinson's disease and neuropsychiatric symptoms. CNS Neurher. 2023;29(8):2259–66. https://doi.org/10.1111/cns.14173. Epub 2023 Mar 16. PMID: 36924300.

4. Noorden V. Medicine is plagued by untrustworthy clinical trials. How many studies are faked or flawed? Nature. 2023;619(7970):454–8. https://doi.org/10.1038/d41586-023-02299-w. PMID: 37464079.
5. Röhner J, Thoss P, Schütz A. Lying on the dissection table: anatomizing faked responses. Behav Res Methods. 2022;54(6):2878–904. https://doi.org/10.3758/s13428-021-01770-8. Epub 2022 Feb 7. PMID: 35132586.

Liver Transplantation: The Recovery of Peter Lichtenstein

36

Charles Troutman

It took two years for Peter Lichtenstein to regain his resolve and get a fresh start at Trinity. Chris knew the details surrounding the deadly epidural case. He was in the hospital that day. Charles Troutman, formerly known as Peter Lichtenstein, changed his name, yet he was unable to find another institution to employ him. His work on the Indian reservation sustained him during these tough times. On the "Office of Medical Conduct" website, the case and the sentence were there. He failed every background check, even though he brought the case up on the few interviews he had. The department backed Peter and voted to have him back in the department when he completed his sentence.

Charles was on the liver transplant anesthesia team. During his leave, a disconnect of communication occurred between the liver transplant anesthesiologists and the surgical transplant team. Chris believed in Charles Troutman and made him Chief of Anesthesia Services for Solid Organ Transplants. Charles was able to reestablish his communication skills for all of the staff on the solid organ transplant team.

The liver transplant team was busier than ever. The national universal problem is that there are shortages of all organs. The organs are allocated by UNOS (United Network of Organ Sharing). The allocations of livers are determined by numerous calculations involving the donor and recipient. The severity of illness of the recipient is in part based on the MELD (Model End Stage Liver Disease) The score estimates how likely a patient is to die from liver disease within three months and is used to determine how urgently a patient needs a liver transplant. The MELD score is based on birthday, bilirubin, sodium, INR, and creatinine. Matching is also based on numerous factors; blood type, transportability, and type of donor.

Donors are categorized into three (or more) pathways. The goal that is shared by all donors is to minimize warm ischemia time. Ideally, a living donor (family or friend) is in an OR at the same hospital as the recipient. A lobe of the liver is removed from the donor and walked over to the recipient's OR. Ischemia time is minimal.

Donation after cardiac death (DCD) is a growing source of organs. A family meets with the transplant team, and all are in agreement that the ongoing decline

C. Scher, *Anesthesia Conversations*,
https://doi.org/10.1007/978-3-032-05354-1_36

and death of their loved one is inevitable. When it is clear that a complete loss of mental status is irreversible, the patient is ready to donate organs. The donor is classified as "donation after cardiac death" (DCD).

The protocol is based on the removal of any tube or catheter that is deemed uncomfortable and is removed in the operating room. This includes extubation. From the time of extubation (beginning of warm ischemia time) to cardiac asystole is everything. If asystole develops in minutes, then the organs can be procured. If the length of time after extubation to asystole is long, warm ischemia time grows and makes the liver less suitable for transplantation. After asystole, there is a "no touch" mandatory 5 min, as patients can auto-resuscitate.

In the "brain dead" patient, the procurement, travel time, and transplant can be timed to minimize warm ischemia time. The number of these ideal donors remains low.

Charles got the call at 8 PM for a transplant from a brain-dead donor to be in the room at 5 AM. Brain death was declared by two independent physicians following a brain-dead protocol. The recipient had a MELD score of 34. He was 67-years-old with long-standing Hepatitis C. His comorbidities included pulmonary hypertension, portal hypertension, portal gastropathy, hepato-renal syndrome, pancytopenia, hyponatremia, bleeding from varices, and hepatic-encephalopathy. There was no evidence of cancer in the liver. The heart of the recipient was hyperdynamic but otherwise fine. The patient started dialysis as soon as the anesthesia team gave them a dialysis line as part of the double-stick technique. The same donor was the source of a new kidney. The donor was 24 years old. Charles's team included a senior resident and a transplant anesthesia fellow.

An RSI was followed by multiple line placements. Charles wanted all lines placed with ultrasound.

The brown port of the triple lumen had a 16-gauge catheter, and both white and blue ports were 18-gauges dedicated for medication administration utilizing the right internal jugular vein. The right internal jugular vein was also cannulated for blood product transfusions and placement of a pulmonary artery catheter. The left internal jugular was dedicated to dialysis if needed. Two arterial lines were needed in case one "went down." A right or left 16-gauge femoral arterial line was placed and checked by both ultrasound and transduction prior to dilation. Ultrasound was needed to prevent repeated blind sticks that could result in a retroperitoneal hemorrhage. The hematocrit would continue to decrease even with a normal surgical field. Despite esophageal varices, it was desirable to have a TEE for hemodynamic management, pulmonary artery pressure measurements, and the response to therapeutics in the pulmonary and systemic vascular beds.

The team planned dialysis throughout this case to maintain potassium levels in a normal range. There is a significant potassium load from the University of Wisconsin Solution and lysed RBCs from the rapid infuser. In a patient who had normal kidney function, dialysis and the dialysis catheter would not have been needed.

On the CT scan, there was no fat visible in the donor liver. There were issues that required critical thinking. The liver was offered to, and rejected by, all of the transplant centers in the UNOS-designated area. If the liver was fatty only under a microscope, it could be used. If the liver appeared yellow, the fat load was too high. With a high MELD score, the patient could die while waiting for a more optimal liver.

The anesthesia team arranged through departmental funds to have point of care testing. The newest version of thromboelastography (TEG) was installed. A PFA (platelet function analyzer), a blood gas machine, and a stat INR device met the needs of the transplant anesthesiologists and surgeons. The PFA's results gave the number of platelets and their function. There is a controversy surrounding the TEG. All residents are now taught that TEG informs the provider which blood products are needed in the bleeding patient.. The TEG has evolved to have readings that are close to real time.

Charles had a different perspective on TEG. He did not want there to be a perfect TEG ever during the transplant. By the end of the first postoperative day, patients become hypercoagulable, and a perfect TEG could enhance clotting in the smallest anastomosis; the critical hepatic artery.

"The surgeons will monitor the hepatic artery with ultrasound countless times in the surgical ICU. If the pulse is lost, it is likely that the patient's hepatic artery is clotted and could need another transplant."

"It does not matter if you believe it or not, this is a colloid case. Bleeding is replaced with blood. When there is no blood available, albumin and hypertonic saline are acceptable bridges to a transfusion solution."

No matter how well a case is proceeding, there is one moment when most patients become unstable hemodynamically. When the liver is "in," and the clamps are released, post-reperfusion syndrome occurs. The release of the portal vein clamp is the most significant unclamping in this syndrome. This is a phenomenon that is not fully understood and is characterized by hypotension, tachycardia, elevation of pulmonary artery pressure, and arrhythmias. The factors that are associated with these changes are metabolic acidosis, hypothermia, ischemia times, fat in the liver, and free radicals. Calcium, Bicarb, epinephrine, and most pressors are administered prophylactically before unclamping. The level of transaminase elevation correlates with the level of injury of hepatocytes.

Hemodynamic stability is assessed by TEE, wedge pressures, and calculations that determine PVR, SVR, and pulse pressure variations. Vasopressin and/or norepinephrine are commonly used as pressors based on the SVR and PVR.

Excellent pain control is achieved only when the patient is intubated. After extubation, pain management becomes challenging. A PCA is not a good choice as encephalopathy is common and takes time to resolve. Charles favored a 15 mg bolus of methadone and titrated remifentanil. Once extubated, Charles favored hydromorphone.

Charles recovered from the epidural case. He was always in the moment and regained his reputation for vigilance, critical thinking and compassion. By five years after the epidural case, most anesthesiologists had only a vague recollection of who the anesthesiologist was for the case.

Suggested Reading

1. Adelmann D, Kronish K, Ramsay MA. Anesthesia for liver transplantation. Anesthesiol Clin. 2017;35(3):491–508. https://doi.org/10.1016/j.anclin.2017.04.006. Epub 2017 Jul 10. PMID: 28784222 Review.
2. Khemichian S, Francoz C, Durand F, Karvellas CJ, Nadim MK. Hepatorenal syndrome. Crit Care Clin. 2021;37(2):321–34. https://doi.org/10.1016/j.ccc.2020.11.011. Epub 2020 Dec 15. PMID: 33752858 Review.
3. Meier RPH, Nunez M, Syed SM, Feng S, Tavakol M, Freise CE, Roberts JP, Ascher NL, Hirose R, Roll GR, et al. Front Immunol. 2023;14:1246867. https://doi.org/10.3389/fimmu.2023.1246867. eCollection 2023. PMID: 37731493.
4. Ruf A, Dirchwolf M, Freeman RB. From Child-Pugh to MELD score and beyond: taking a walk down memory lane. Ann Hepatol. 2022;27(1):100535. https://doi.org/10.1016/j.aohep.2021.100535. Epub 2021 Sep 22. PMID: 34560316.
5. Tapper EB, Parikh ND. Diagnosis and management of cirrhosis and its complications: a review. JAMA. 2023;329(18):1589–602. https://doi.org/10.1001/jama.2023.5997. PMID: 37159031 Review.
6. Vasant Kulkarni S, Rao PP, Naidu CS, Pathak N, Singh AK. Evaluation of implantable Doppler probe continuous monitoring of hepatic artery anastomosis after liver transplantation. Med J Armed Forces India. 2021;77(3):349–54. https://doi.org/10.1016/j.mjafi.2020.03.012. Epub 2020 Jun 3. PMID: 34305290.
7. Vidgren M, Oniscu GC. Liver transplantation from uncontrolled DCD donors – is there light at the end of the tunnel? Liver Transpl. 2024;30(1):6–7. https://doi.org/10.1097/LVT.0000000000000267. Epub 2023 Sep 29. PMID: 37773027.

Anesthesia for Carcinoid Syndrome

37

Jen Davis

Jen started to decline when she was 15. She was considered the "smartest kid" by her fellow students in high school. Her essays were always prolific, and her cursive writing was better than that in instruction books. She had been an activist for female-related issues whether it was equal pay, pro-choice, and access to quality employment. Jen's family was more than supportive and loving, and from a glance, her life was soaring.

During January of the first year of high school, something went awry. She was admitted to Touro Hospital for bulimia. Her hair always looked like it needed to be washed, and her choice of clothing was all too tight to accentuate a false image of her body. She withdrew from her social network that was, at one time, huge. Her diagnosis was Anorexia Nervosa.

Jen's parents were frantic and extremely concerned and frightened. They did their homework to find a psychologist and psychiatrist. It is unusual to have more than one serious diagnosis in medicine. Anorexia Nervosa did seem to fit. She lost a sense of reality concerning her body image. When sitting in a chair, she would rock back and forth just to burn calories. At Thanksgiving, she would fill her plate with the usual savory dishes and secretly go to the bathroom and stick a finger down her throat to induce vomiting. Her teeth had turned brown years ago from the staining of her enamel from gastric acid bathing her teeth.

Jen was admitted to a psychiatric hospital while in the middle of the 11th grade. With a team of psychiatrists, psychologists, social workers, and nutritionists, Jen's weight stabilized. Jen found true bonding in group therapy and actually gained weight. Her goal was 100 pounds from 86 pounds. Under great duress, she made her goal weight. The threat of tube feeding through her nose was a wake-up call to see that her illness was going to kill her. After 3 months of treatment, Jen understood her illness, and while there would be setbacks, she was finally on the right path.

Her college life at Tulane improved her self-perception. She had developed into an attractive young woman who rediscovered socialization and friendships. With excellent nutrition, she finished her second year weighing 110 pounds. Her teeth were not

C. Scher, *Anesthesia Conversations*,
https://doi.org/10.1007/978-3-032-05354-1_37

salvageable, and with implants and veneers. She appeared normal the work of the state-of-the-art cosmetic dentists was transformative in giving Jen a beautiful smile.

Jen's sense of fashion was suitable for a college student: tight jeans, flip-flops, and T-shirts. She was happy with her body and finally "fit in" with the fashion of the college world. Jen had some degree of peace of mind and upped her game by joining a sorority. For the first time in her life, she had devoted friends. She was able to organize her academic life. With all that she went through, she was inspired to be a psychiatrist or psychologist.

It was time. Jen wanted to divulge her eating disorder to her close sorority sisters. The subject would come up, and she wanted to divulge her illness to her friends. She was right in believing they would rescue her when she reverted to her eating disorder. With her growing confidence, she was ready to date.

Drew Lowry was a classmate whom Jen did not know. He always sat a few seats from Jen in the classes they shared: cell biology, chemistry, and history. Drew was hell bent on going to medical school and rarely took some time off from his manic study schedule. He stepped out of his world and asked Jen out for coffee.

Jen was thrilled, but feared that she would not be able to hold it together with the calories of a scone or muffin. Jen was grateful that it was coffee and not going to a bar to drink something much stronger. She had never had alcohol in her life and wanted to give it a shot alone in her apartment. After saying yes to Drew, she started to over think the date. She was always too sick to consider a date. She never had sex, not even a kiss. Would she be capable of having the tumultuous swings of having a boyfriend? She was and she did.

In her third year at Tulane, Jen had her first asthmatic attack. She was treated at Tulane with albuterol and was sent home with budesonide/glycopyrrolate/formoterol fumarate. Jen's asthma was in check for six months until she woke up one morning in severe respiratory distress. She was frightened and air hungry in the emergency department at Tulane. The results of her arterial blood gas prompted a STAT page for anesthesia. With a CO_2 of 74 and an O_2 of 68, Jen needed mechanical ventilation.

Jen was intubated with a rapid sequence induction: ketamine and double-dose rocuronium. She was transported to the ICU with an infusion of propofol for sedation.

She spent 48 h on a ventilator in the ICU and spent 2 more days on nasal oxygen. Rounds in the ICU included medical students, critical care fellows, anesthesia residents, and her nurses. What started as a discharge discussion evolved into a major breakthrough discussion led by a medical student. The student combed through Jen's chart. No one was aware that Jen had made four visits over the last two weeks to the emergency room for horrific diarrhea. The student strongly suggested that Jen had Carcinoid Syndrome. The critical care fellow arranged for a PET scan.

PET scans, particularly Ga-68 Dotatate PET/CT, stage carcinoid tumors, FDG PET Gallium-68 Dotatate uses a radioactive tracer that binds to somatostatin receptors on carcinoid cells. This allows, for better visualization of tumors and their metastases.

Blood was drawn for chromogranin, and urine was collected for 24 h to measure 5-HIAA. GI was consulted for upper endoscopy and colonoscopy, followed by a pulmonary consult for a possible bronchoscopy.

An infusion of octreotide (somatostatin) was started immediately after Jen's pulmonary status stabilized. The somatostatins inhibit the release of serotonin from the tumor. The hunt was on to determine the location of the carcinoid tumor. There was no disease in the liver. The PET scan was consistent with the finding of the carcinoid tumor in the small intestine by endoscopy and in the lungs determined by bronchoscopy. There was no disease in the liver.

A surgical consult favored a small bowel resection, lung resection, and somatostatin analogs. Octreotide or Telotristat, reduce the production of serotonin in the body. They are weaned down after resection of carcinoid tumors. These drugs are used in combination with a somatostatin analog to control diarrhea associated with carcinoid syndrome.

Jen was on the schedule for resection of the small bowel and a tumor in the lung. There had to be more tumors that did not appear on imaging at the time. These micrometastastases could be held in check. The first part of the surgery was to resect the lung tumor. The case would be done by a minimally invasive approach. The colorectal surgeons would deal with the bowel. The tumor load would be lessened, and symptoms could disappear or be mild.

Jen was extubated in the operating room. She was breathing comfortably, and her abdominal pain was controllable. She asked if she was cured. The answer to her question was a challenge to explain. Cure comes if the lung and small bowel are the only parts of the body involved. With a surveillance schedule, other locations could be addressed immediately. Six months after the initial surgery, Jen felt well.

With a lifetime of chaos with her health, she was able to generate a GPA and USMLE score that fit right in with most of the medical schools in the country. She felt the need to stay in New Orleans, where her doctors were. Every medical student in New Orleans knew the legendary duo of Chris and Lily. Jen made an appointment with Lily and was given a spot in the Trinity School of Medicine after a 20-minute discussion. Chris and Lily kept tabs on Jena to be sure that she was well and getting the education that she wanted. Lily mentored Jen in the process of discovery that led to the selection of a career. Jen was all in for an anesthesia residency and a critical care fellowship.

Chris's reputation for having the back of everyone in the department was all she needed to hear. While she wanted to be deployed to the surgical ICU 100% of her clinical time, Chris thought that she should spend some time in the OR, and then he changed his mind. Jen could be 100% in the ICU.

Chris was not successful in building a critical care team. Jen was the only critical care attending that he recruited. Jen found a friend at a sorority reunion in New Orleans who was a Critical Care Attending at Jackson Memorial in Miami. Chris let Jen do the recruiting. Chris gave Jen an itinerary to follow when Gabriella arrived. Jen discovered three additional critical care attendings. Chris did all of the hotel and restaurant reservations. He gave Jen his credit card in case she needed it.

Jen remained asymptomatic for the rest of her life. Surgery "cured" her. Initially, she gave blood and urine samples every 6 months for 5 years. The surveillance was deemed to be over for the rest of her life. Chris was always supportive and gave Jen every resource she needed.

After 20 years as an attending in the surgical ICU, Jen switched gears and completed a one-year fellowship in Public Health. Her new career allowed her more time with her husband, Drew, and their four children. Jen leaned heavily on the support of her therapists, who were a must for the rest of her life.

Suggested Reading

1. Ammann M, Kinney MAO, Gudmundsdottir H, Santol J, Thiels CA, Warner SG, Truty MJ, Kendrick ML, Smoot RL, Anderson AL, Halfdanarson TR, Nagorney DM, Starlinger PP. Comparison of octreotide and vasopressors as first-line treatment for intraoperative carcinoid crisis. Ann Surg Oncol. 2024;31(6):3976–7. https://doi.org/10.1245/s10434-024-15264-2. Epub 2024 Apr 15.
2. Castillo M, Weiselberg E. Bulimia nervosa/purging disorder. Curr Probl Pediatr Adolesc Health Care. 2017;47(4):85–94. https://doi.org/10.1016/j.cppeds.2017.02.004. PMID: 28532966 Review.
3. Ito T, Lee L, Jensen RT. Carcinoid-syndrome: recent advances, current status and controversies. Curr Opin Endocrinol Diabetes Obes. 2018;25(1):22–35. https://doi.org/10.1097/MED.0000000000000376. PMID: 29120923.
4. Robelin P, Hadoux J, Forestier J, Planchard D, Hervieu V, Berdelou A, Scoazec JY, Valette PJ, Leboulleux S, Ducreux M, Lombard-Bohas C, Baudin E, Walter T. Characterization, prognosis, and treatment of patients with metastatic lung carcinoid tumors. J Thorac Oncol. 2019;14(6):993–1002. https://doi.org/10.1016/j.jtho.2019.02.002. Epub 2019 Feb 13. PMID: 30771520.
5. Uniacke B, Walsh BT. Eating disorders. Ann Intern Med. 2022;175(8):ITC113–28. https://doi.org/10.7326/AITC202208160. Epub 2022 Aug 9. PMID: 35939813 Review.

Anesthesia for Paraganglioma/ Pheochromocytoma

38

Iris Goldsmith

Some lives are simply smitten. Before she purchased the robotic glove, Iris trained her affected hand to do many of the anesthesia procedures one-handed. While she had a system for each procedure, her ability to do tasks was not as fast as she needed.

Five years after the stroke, she developed severe symptoms in her body that were more than alarming. Most of her symptoms were nonspecific, including headaches, palpitations, sweating, anxiety, nervousness, abdominal pain, nausea, fatigue, dizziness, intolerance to heat, paresthesias, pain, blurred vision, and diarrhea. Most of her symptoms were mild, but her anxiety could not be higher.

Chris had a friend who was an endocrine surgeon at Trinity. Iris had an appointment with Dr. Rubin. Vital signs were taken, and shockingly, her blood pressure was 210/95. Her pulse was 100, and there was a low-grade fever of 38.1. Iris asked to run to the bathroom. She had diarrhea with urgency that started with abdominal cramps four days ago.

Dr. Rubin entered the room, and Iris was now fearful. He was sure that her symptoms were due to excessive catecholamines. Blood was drawn for metanephrines and normetanephrines. The results would be back the next day. As suspected by Dr. Rubin, Iris had either the classical pheochromocytoma or a metanephrine secreting paraganglioma.

The blood metanephrines and normetanephrines in Iris were significantly elevated. The PET-CT demonstrated a large paraganglioma with a blood supply coming from the aorta. The scan was significant for the tumor, which is all white on the PET scan. The "whiteness" was interpreted as a highly vascular tumor.

The PET scan did not reveal any other location for neuroendocrine tumors. A transthoracic echo demonstrated a profound cardiomyopathy with an ejection fraction of 25%. The heart was overworking against the increased afterload caused by the excess catecholamines.

"The standard of care for the preparation for surgery is to initiate alpha blockade with doxazosin or any drug in that family. There are those clinicians who alpha

C. Scher, *Anesthesia Conversations*,
https://doi.org/10.1007/978-3-032-05354-1_38

block for seven to ten days followed by beta blockade. There is a wide range of practice from no preparation to a conservative practice that Dr. Rubin followed. He used nadolol for beta blockade. He waited until the blood pressure was less than 140/90 and stable before surgery.

Care for neuroendocrine tumors has evolved and changed preop- preparation. The ICU is not necessary for the management of blood pressures. Most cases are laparoscopic with one night in the hospital. If the blood pressure is trending down, there is no reason to stay in the hospital. There are extreme cases when hypertension does not resolve, and the ejection fraction is less than 25%., A laparotomy maybe needed to hunt down more than one endocrine tumor in the patient."

Iris's case lasted 90 min. Her first blood pressure in the PACU was 132/85. Her discharge pressure was 128/83. All of her symptoms that were attributed to her excess of catecholamines resolved within days.

Did Chris have a knack for hiring so many people with personal problems? Chris would say that you cannot find any group of people where 50% of any group have less personal problems.

Iris was born and raised in Kazakhstan and came to Philadelphia with her family when she was 15. She went to Penn State for college, Thomas Jefferson for medical School, and Virgina Mason for her Regional Anesthesia Fellowship. She came to live in New Orleans after three consecutive years of attending Jazz Fest. Her neurological deficits from her stroke did not improve.

Suggested Reading

1. Carrasquillo JA, Chen CC, Jha A, Ling A, Lin FI, Pryma DA, Pacak K. Imaging of pheochromocytoma and paraganglioma. J Nucl Med. 2021;62(8):1033–42. https://doi.org/10.2967/jnumed.120.259689. PMID: 34330739.
2. Fang F, Ding L, He Q, Liu M. Preoperative management of pheochromocytoma and paraganglioma. Front Endocrinol (Lausanne). 2020;11:586795. https://doi.org/10.3389/fendo.2020.586795. eCollection 2020.
3. Farrugia FA, Charalampopoulos A. Pheochromocytoma. Endocr Regul. 2019;53(3):191–212. https://doi.org/10.2478/enr-2019-0020. PMID: 31517632.
4. Lenders JW, Duh QY, Eisenhofer G, Gimenez-Roqueplo AP, Grebe SK, Murad MH, Naruse M, Pacak K, Young WF Jr. Pheochromocytoma and paraganglioma: an endocrine society clinical practice guideline. J Clin Endocrinol Metab. 2014;99(6):1915–42. https://doi.org/10.1210/jc.2014-1498. PMID: 24893135.
5. Leung K, Stamm M, Raja A, Low G. Pheochromocytoma: the range of appearances on ultrasound, CT, MRI, and functional imaging. AJR Am J Roentgenol. 2013;200(2):370–8. https://doi.org/10.2214/AJR.12.9126.
6. Wang K, Crona J, Beuschlein F, Grossman AB, Pacak K, Nölting S. Targeted therapies in pheochromocytoma and paraganglioma. J Clin Endocrinol Metab. 2022;107(11):2963–72. https://doi.org/10.1210/clinem/dgac471. PMID: 35973976.
7. Yip L, Duh QY, Wachtel H, Jimenez C, Sturgeon C, Lee C, Velázquez-Fernández D, Berber E, Hammer GD, Bancos I, Lee JA, Marko J, Morris-Wiseman LF, Hughes MS, Livhits MJ, Han MA, Smith PW, Wilhelm S, Asa SL, Fahey TJ 3rd, McKenzie TJ, Strong VE, Perrier ND. American Association of Endocrine Surgeons Guidelines for Adrenalectomy: executive summary. JAMA Surg. 2022;157(10):870–7. https://doi.org/10.1001/jamasurg.2022.3544.

Alpha-1-Antitrypsin Deficiency

39

Kevin McBride

Kevin McBride was born a block from the unloading docks on the Thames. His parents worked the docks and were salt of the earth, except that they were bad drunks. Kevin always had a shiner in one or both of his eyes, cigarette burns on his back, and the gait of an old man. By age 7, he still had not been enrolled in a school. His parents could not make it happen.

Kevin's best friend was Carter. They met playing soccer in an alley near the river. Carter was mature beyond his years and sensed there was something disturbing in Kevin's life. Kevin's clothing was filthy, and he was desperately in need of a bath. Carter revealed to his parents Kevin's situation and immediately called the DfE (Department for Education).

The Department for Education (DfE) is responsible for child protection in England. It sets out policy, legislation, and statutory guidance on how the child protection system should work.

It makes clear the expectations and requirements around the duties of care to children and creates accountability for these. The main legislation in England includes the Children Act 1989, the Children Act 2004, and the Children and Social Work Act 2017.

The officials arrived at Carter's home and notified Kevin's parents that Kevin was in the process of moving him out of harm's way and placing him in a "safe haven." Kevin's family did not resist at all and were clearly both drunk. Kevin gave Carter a fist pump. Kevin suddenly became weepy. His tears were not about his parents. He was finally done with the beatings and verbal abuse. Carter's parents offered to take Kevin in and adopt him as a son. Kevin just wanted some space and time and declined the offer. The issue was not closed, and Kevin ultimately conceded. He was adopted, and brother Kevin's survival skills were no longer needed.

It was a struggle at first, but Kevin was able to catch up to the second graders. He was only one year behind Carter, and Kevin was clearly bright. He studied for tests

C. Scher, *Anesthesia Conversations*,
https://doi.org/10.1007/978-3-032-05354-1_39

and had intellectual curiosity that is usually identified at an older age. A trip to the library always made his day.

Carter's parents, Clifford and Mary, were well known as prosecutors. Their seamless characters and work ethic earned them admission to the London School of Economics and Political Science. After their marriage, they both served as barristers in London for the rest of their working lives. Mary took some time off to put Carter on the path of having a sustainable career. Carter chose medicine. Kevin was a mirror image of Carter in terms of academic achievement and also chose medicine

The boys were heavily influenced by the opinions of Cliff and Mary. Cliff wanted the boys to get their medical degree in the United States. The only medical school that Kevin was accepted to was Trinity, while Carter was accepted to Northwestern, Dartmouth, Columbia, NYU, and Trinity.

Chris used his "power" to have the Dean of the School of Medicine make sure both boys went to medical school at Trinity. Lily kept tabs on the brothers and would offer them an out-of-the-match position in Lily's anesthesia residency. It was an unspoken fact that Kevin and Carter had to be in the same anesthesia training program.

At the end of the first medical school semester, Kevin complained of severe fatigue with weight loss. Carter knew there was something really wrong with Kevin. Their health insurance was covered by Trinity. Carter asked the Dean to recommend a boarded Professor of Internal Medicine. Dr. Ellen Dubois was now in charge of Kevin's case.

Ten tubes of blood were drawn, and the turnaround time for most of the labs was an hour. The boys went for some coffee in the cafeteria while waiting for the results. Kevin's phone rang, but he did not change the settings, and all phone calls went straight to voicemail. The content of the voicemail was impossible to decipher, but the doctor's voice was almost somber.

Kevin's white cell count was over 100,000. Kevin knew enough that he had some form of leukemia. The doctor arranged a bone marrow aspirate and biopsy.

Kevin had acute myelocytic leukemia and was devastated. He was admitted for further workup and treatment. His bone marrow was resistant to chemotherapy and immunotherapy. A harrowing bone marrow transplant was successful. Kevin endured graft versus host disease, sepsis, and jaundice, which all resolved in time. He progressed to "Clinical Remission."

After a year spent on treatment, he was ready to restart medical school at Trinity. Kevin agreed to the Dean's request. He needed to start medical school again. Kevin was appreciative of that opportunity and outworked all of his classmates. Carter was entering his internship, and Kevin was a fourth-year medical student. For the first time, the boys were separated and now were responsible for their own decisions.

Carter completed his anesthesia residency and went back to live in the UK. There was reciprocity between the UK and USA physicians with some hurdles. Carter practiced anesthesiology at London Bridge Hospital.

During his fourth year of medical school, Kevin developed shortness of breath, weight loss, jaundice, and was physically impaired. He could not walk up a flight of stairs without extreme shortness of breath. Dr. Dubois recommended Dr. Jacob

Lukin, Chief of Hepatology. She arranged an appointment for Kevin ASAP. Dr. Lukin wanted to see Kevin now!

Kevin was directly admitted to the medical ICU for dyspnea and jaundice. On exam, Kevin was jaundiced, gaunt, and wheezing at a level that you could hear without a stethoscope. His vital signs were a blood pressure of 70/40, heart rate of 120 beats per minute, temperature of 38.5, respiratory rate of 20, and an oxygen saturation of 88%. Dr. Lukin ordered an albuterol treatment and intravenous fluids while waiting for the results of Keven's blood tests and a CT scan of the chest and abdomen.

Kevin was declining quickly and was visibly air hungry. Anesthesia was called for an intubation, a central line, and an arterial line. Kevin was sedated with low-dose propofol and dexmedetomidine and norepinephrine at 10 mcg an hour to support his blood pressure.

His CT scan of his lungs was significant for severe COPD and pneumonia. The CT of the abdomen revealed a cirrhotic liver. It was now clear that Kevin had alpha-1-antitrypsin deficiency. The lab results came back in one hour. Kevin's liver ALT was three times normal. His significantly elevated bilirubin was expected.

Alpha-1-antitrypsin (AAT) is a polyfunctional protein that inhibits neutrophil elastase, whose function is the proteolytic degradation of matrix proteins. Genetic deficiency of AAT results in an imbalance in activity between the proteinase and the anti-proteinase (AAT). This imbalance leads to the breakdown of elastin in tissues in the parenchyma of the lung. Abnormal AAT proteins build up in the liver, causing cirrhosis.

It is likely that a family member had a subclinical case, or there may have been a mutation that prevented the expression of the protein. There is no information about Kevin's parents. It is essential to determine the involvement of the liver and lungs. After imaging and biopsies, Kevin's liver MELD (bilirubin, creatinine, and INR) score was 32. His score puts him on the high liver transplant waiting list.

Several spirometry tests, DLCO, and lung biopsy demonstrated severe COPD. Infusions of alpha-1-antitrypsin could stop or slow down the advancement of lung disease by adding alpha-1-antitrypsin to the lungs. Ensifentrine is a PDE3/4 inhibitor (phosphodiesterase inhibitor) that "calms lung inflammation." This medical management improved Kevin's pulmonary status dramatically. He underwent a liver transplant without any significant pulmonary complications. He would not need a lung transplant in his life.

Suggested Reading

1. Casas F, Blanco I, et al. Indications for active case searches and intravenous alpha-1 antitrypsin treatment for patients with alpha-1 antitrypsin deficiency chronic pulmonary obstructive disease: an update. Arch Bronconeumol. 2015;51(4):185–92. https://doi.org/10.1016/j.arbres.2014.05.008. Epub 2014 Jul 12.
2. Dasí F. Alpha-1 antitrypsin deficiency. Med Clin (Barc). 2023;160(5):203–5. https://doi.org/10.1016/j.medcli.2022.09.001. Epub 2022 Oct 14. PMID: 36253208.

3. Lechowicz U, Rudzinski S, Jezela-Stanek A, Janciauskiene S, Chorostowska-Wynimko J. Post-translational modifications of circulating alpha-1-antitrypsin protein. Int J Mol Sci. 2020;21(23):9187. https://doi.org/10.3390/ijms21239187. PMID: 3327.
4. McElvaney OF, Fraughen DD, McElvaney OJ, Carroll TP, McElvaney NG. Alpha-1 antitrypsin deficiency: current therapy and emerging targets. Expert Rev Respir Med. 2023;17(3):191–202. https://doi.org/10.1080/17476348.2023.2174973. Epub 2023 Mar 15. PMID: 36.
5. Pires Ferreira D, Gruntman AM, Flotte TR. Gene therapy for alpha-1 antitrypsin deficiency: an update. Expert Opin Biol Ther. 2023;23(3):283–91. https://doi.org/10.1080/14712598.2023.2183771. Epub 2023 Mar 2. PMID: 36825473.
6. Stockley RA, Turner AM. Alpha-1-antitrypsin deficiency: clinical variability, assessment, and treatment. Trends Mol Med. 2014;20(2):105–15. https://doi.org/10.1016/j.molmed.2013.11.006. Epub 2013 Dec 28. PMID: 24380646.
7. Wewers MD, Crystal RG. Alpha-1 antitrypsin augmentation therapy. COPD. 2013;10(Suppl 1):64–7. https://doi.org/10.3109/15412555.2013.764402. PMID: 23527997.

Prolonged QT Interval and Cardiac Arrest

40

Sofia Gangliono

Lauren arranged a monthly "Girls Night Out." The females in the department met monthly at the "Napoleon House" for drinks and conversation with a touch of raunchiness to it. In the first hour at the bar, Sofia had three martinis and a Bloody Mary. There were no signs of inebriation, which substantiated her legacy as being a well-controlled drunk.

Sofia took two sips of her fifth drink and then collapsed to the floor. She did nothing to break her fall. The entire table was in shock and did a quick evaluation. She was apneic and asystolic. Lauran called 911, and everyone participated in cardiopulmonary resuscitation. Each member took turns delivering 100 compressions per minute for two minutes and then switching for relief. There was an AED in the restaurant, and Irene took the lead by calling out the steps of resuscitation.

The pads for an EKG and defibrillation were attached. Sofia was asystolic and in a non-shockable rhythm. After 15 more minutes of CPR, EMS arrived. The EKG remained flatline. Lauren continued CPR with 100 compressions per minute. EMT placed an IV and administered 1 mg of epinephrine, which had no impact. Chest compressions continued. Iris took a laryngoscope from the EMS pack and intubated without disrupting CPR.

The plan was to get Sofia on a spine board to transfer her to the ambulance without a prolonged break in CPR. Lara gave a second dose of epinephrine without any change in her asystolic heart rhythm. Lily made a reasonable suggestion to manually shock Sofia in case the EKG revealed fine ventricular fibrillation and not asystole.

With minimal disruption of CPR, Sofia was loaded onto the ambulance, and a member of the EMS team put a cervical collar on as she did nothing to break her fall. The EMS driver grabbed Sofia's purse, inspected the contents, and saw vials for quetiapine, lamictal, and klonopin. The klonopin and lamictal vials had 60 pills in each. The 500 mg quetiapine vial was empty!

C. Scher, *Anesthesia Conversations*,
https://doi.org/10.1007/978-3-032-05354-1_40

Irene opened the electronic record in the Emergency room and easily found Sofia's medical chart. There were multiple EKGs in the cardiology section. Sofia had a significantly prolonged QT interval.

"Why would they put her on quetiapine with a chart that documented a prolonged QT interval?"

" Quetiapine, which can have a prolonged QT on top of Sofia's baseline long QT, tipped her over to Toursades de Pointes followed by asystole. Why don't psychiatrists get a baseline QT interval before they start a patient on an atypical antipsychotic. If not, why not!" Irene was befuddled.

The ambulance took 8 min to arrive from the bar to the Trinity Emergency room. Irene accompanied Sofia in the ambulance and paged the chief resident of anesthesia to bring a bag of intralipid to the ED.

Intralipid has a long history of success with overdoses of psychiatric medications besides local anesthetic toxicity. CPR continued, and only Iris had experience with intralipid. The dose of 20% intralipid was 1.5 mg/kg lean body mass. Within 3 min after the intralipid infusion, Sofia was able to breathe on her own. Her femoral pulse was strong, and her heart rate was in sinus rhythm. Her blood pressure needed support with low-dose norepinephrine. Sofia's pupils were reactive to light, and her patellar tendon reflex was brisk.

There was a bed in the MICU, and Sofia spent a night on a ventilator. She needed no sedation due to the quetiapine. Everyone expected her to make a full recovery. By morning, she was arousable and bucking on the endotracheal tube. Lauren went to the ICU the next morning. Sophia was alert and was extubated.

It was expected that Sofia would have a significant withdrawal from the quetiapine and needed a supervised detox. They would start her on her normal dose and wean her down. She never, in years, had a problem with the quetiapine. It was the whole bottle that did her in. She objected to the wean. There was no reason. She had been fine with the 500 mg dose.

When Sofia woke up, the Chairman of Psychiatry was now her doctor. Sofia's bipolar disease was more about mania superimposed on a baseline high-energy state. The booze was to knock down the energy level. It is easier to deal with mania than depression. She denied that she ever had depression. Her psychiatrist corrected Sofia. How is an overdose not a symptom of depression?

Her suicide attempt was based on bipolar depression. She was sure that her colleagues knew of her diagnosis and thought she should not be practicing medicine. There was no truth to that perception. Her psychiatrist knew that her colleagues were aware of her diagnosis for years. They loved her and thought she was a brilliant doctor who was essential to the team. Her psychiatrist put her on an antidepressant, which could be problematic for a bipolar patient whose tendency is hypomania.

Chris made Sofia take some time off to get her back to her baseline. Chris put Sofia on leave with no deadline. She would return to work when her psychiatrist gave her clearance. Sofia's burden of keeping her diagnosis private was over. The entire department was sure that Sofia was bipolar for years, simply from her behavior. Bipolar Sofia was treated by her friends and colleagues with dignity and respect for the rest of her career.

Suggested Reading

1. Beach SR, Celano CM, Noseworthy PA, Januzzi JL, Huffman JC. QTc prolongation, torsades de pointes, and psychotropic medications. Psychosomatics. 2013;54(1):1–13. https://doi.org/10.1016/j.psym.2012.11.001. PMID: 23295003
2. Lee SH, Sohn JT. Mechanisms underlying lipid emulsion resuscitation for drug toxicity: a narrative review. Korean J Anesthesiol. 2023;76(3):171–82. https://doi.org/10.4097/kja.23031. Epub 2023 Jan 26. PMID: 36704816.
3. Miller JN, Black DW. Bipolar disorder and suicide: a review. Curr Psychiatry Rep. 2020;22(2):6. https://doi.org/10.1007/s11920-020-1130-0. PMID: 31955273.
4. Sher L, Oquendo MA. Suicide: an overview for clinicians. Clin North Am. 2023;107(1):119–30. https://doi.org/10.1016/j.mcna.2022.03.008. Epub 2022 Oct 28. PMID: 36402494.

41 Bilateral Stellate Ganglion Blocks for Atrial Fibrillation

Esther David

Esther rinsed her razor and placed it in the medicine cabinet in the same spot as always. She started to shave her head the day after she married a stranger. They were a Hasidic couple where the men studied the Talmud and other Jewish liturgy while the women had some secular education. The role of a woman included bearing children, keeping house, and being subservient to her husband. Her husband had a cash business which he kept secret from Esther. She had no idea what he did and was afraid to ask.

Esther David, who married at 19, was a victim of spousal abuse, both verbal and physical. There was never a time that she could remember that she did not have a black eye, a missing front tooth, and bruises all over her body. Sex was never consensual and resembled a rape. This was "par for the course" in the community and was a secret to any family and friends. Abuse was part of the culture, and Esther wanted out. She was never pregnant. Esther was good at keeping records of her periods and knew when she was not fertile. She wanted to escape and planned her departure without a soul having any knowledge of her wishes.

Esther had never been in a subway, bus, or taxi. She made a detailed map for her departure. She rarely saw her husband during Shabbat. Her escape day would be next Saturday. While her husband gave her cash to shop for food, she did not have any extra money. She knew exactly where her husband hid the money. There were 2000 dollars in one of his versions of the Talmud. A rectangle was carved out in the middle of the book. She estimated that there was a total of 10,000 in the bank. Esther took the 2000 dollars and fled.

Esther had a fifth-grade education. She did not want to start her new life in the fifth grade of a public elementary school. She had no money, skills, or a single friend who could help her. She blindly walked into a reform temple and met with the rabbi. Coincidentally, the rabbi had a long history of helping women escape from their Hasidic life.

"Please go to a 'Footsteps' meeting." Footsteps is a New York-based organization that provides support resources for women who want to leave the Hasidic

C. Scher, *Anesthesia Conversations*,
https://doi.org/10.1007/978-3-032-05354-1_41

community. Footsteps offers services to make the transition into secular life. Members can discuss educational scholarships and connect with volunteers, education coaches, and peer study buddies. They can obtain resources to navigate educational settings. Esther applied and was accepted each year for funding of her education that included tutors, digital literacy, and computers.

It was arranged that Esther would live with another woman who also fled the Hasidic life. She was able to earn enough money to live off from part-time jobs. Her education was provided by tutors. She did not have to be embarrassed in public starting at the fifth grade. She was connected to multiple tutors. From the time she entered school until she graduated with a GED took 10 years. She was accepted to the City College of New York and was able to achieve grades that were accepted by many medical schools. Her path over 20 years was the subject of the New Yorker.

Esther applied to 100 medical schools and was accepted to Sackler New York State, located in Tel Aviv, Israel. The school was recognized as a United States medical school. She was accepted to one anesthesia residency: Trinity. Esther David became a faculty member at the age of 50.

A 52-year-old male was transferred from Memorial Hospital to Trinity for treatment of refractory atrial fibrillation. His medical history was otherwise normal. He presented to the Memorial ED with heart palpitations that started six months ago. An EKG confirmed the diagnosis of atrial fibrillation. His ventricular response rate was 122 with a blood pressure of 137/90. Due to his stable vital signs, no cardioversion was attempted. Five milligrams of metoprolol lowered the ventricular heart rate of 88. The patient was discharged with flecainide, amiodarone, apixaban, a Zio patch, and an appointment in one week at the cardiology clinic. The patient inquired about the Zio patch. It is a small adhesive patch that monitors heart rhythm for 2 weeks.

While the cardiology team ordered Flecainide and Amiodarone, it was viewed as a temporary fix. Long-term use of flecainide could cause coronary artery disease or structural damage to the heart. Long-term use of amiodarone could lead to pulmonary fibrosis. The cardiologists had great concerns of anticoagulation for a 52 year old for the rest of her life.

At a clinic visit, the patient was comfortable, in normal sinus rhythm but was out of breath more than he should be from a walk from the parking garage to the clinic. The patient was in normal sinus rhythm, The Zio patch was interpreted as the patient was in atrial fibrillation 45% of the time.

An echocardiogram explained dyspnea on mild exertion. The ejection fraction was 20% The myocardium was globally hypokinetic. Valvular function was normal. A nuclear PET stress test was read as diffuse cardiac ischemia not amenable to stenting.

The diagnosis now included chronic congestive heart failure and atrial fibrillation. The patient consented to an AICD (automatic implantable cardioverter defibrillator) followed by an atrial fibrillation ablation on the following day.

The A-fib ablation was successful, but a return of atrial fibrillation was always possible. The need for anticoagulation was resolved with the placement of a

Watchman, a device inserted into the left atrial appendage. The Watchman served as a "net" for blood clots that form stasis of blood in the heart during atrial fibrillation.

The patient tolerated the procedures without complication. The medications originally prescribed, except for apixaban, were continued. Entresto was added to unload the heart for chronic CHF.

Two weeks after the AICD implant, the patient entered the Emergency Department. His chief complaint was nothing more than " I feel like I have Covid."

His vital signs were normal except for his temperature, which was 38.6. The Covid test was negative. The metabolic blood tests were normal, but his CBC was not. The white cell count was 18,000 with a left shift. The patient was treated for an infected AICD. The AICD was removed, and a two-week course of antibiotics was ordered.

An echocardiogram revealed clots in both left and right atria. An EKG was consistent with the return of atrial fibrillation with a ventricular response of 137. A block of the sympathetic output to the heart could keep the deleterious effects of a rapid ventricular response at bay. Esther David offered the electrophysiology cardiologists a bilateral stellate ganglion block. The blocks would eliminate the sympathetic output that drives most tachyarrhythmias. Esther David, from the Department of Anesthesiology, was consulted to perform the block. The blocks last up to 72 h. Two blocks were planned before a new AICD was inserted.

Stellate ganglion blocks are performed for the management of patients for a variety of pain conditions, including complex regional pain syndrome, peripheral vascular disease, and cardiac tachyarrhythmias. Employing ultrasound, the bilateral block took 20 min. The patient's rhythm after the blocks was a normal sinus rhythm. A second set of blocks were performed six days after the first one, allowing the full course of antibiotics needed. There were no episodes of tachyarrhythmias.

Another mapping with an ablation was successful. A new AICD was placed the following day. The next cardiology clinic appointment was in six months. Esther's clinical reputation soared in the electrophysiology department, and a piece of her past life was disappearing.

Suggested Reading

1. Chouairi F, Rajkumar K, Benak A, Qadri Y, Piccini JP, Mathew J, Ray ND, Toman J, Kautzner J, Ganesh A, Sramko M, Fudim M. A multicenter study of stellate ganglion block as a temporizing treatment for refractory ventricular arrhythmias. JACC Clin Electrophysiol. 2024;10(4):750–8. https://doi.org/10.1016/j.jacep.2023.12.012. Epub 2024 Feb 14. PMID: 38363278.
2. Ganesh A, Qadri YJ, Boortz-Marx RL, Al-Khatib SM, Harpole DH Jr, Katz JN, Koontz JI, Mathew JP, Ray ND, Sun AY, Tong BC, Ulloa L, Piccini JP, Fudim M. Stellate ganglion blockade: an intervention for the management of ventricular arrhythmias. Curr Hypertens Rep. 2020;22(12):100. https://doi.org/10.1007/s11906-020-01111-8. PMID: 33097982.
3. Glaberson W. Orthodox Jews battle neighbors in a zoning war, New York Times, June 3, 1991, at Al ("The motivation of some people is that they do not want the Ultra-Orthodox or the Hasidim to move in.").
4. LeBlanc-Sternberg v. Fletcher, 781 E Supp. 261,264 (S.D.N.Y. 1991).

5. Runyon v. McCrary 427 U.S. 160, 169 n. 8, (1976) (stating that a "portion" of the Civil Rights Act of 1866 is presently codified in 42 U.S.C. § 1981); Jones v. Alfred H. Mayer Co., 392 U.S. 409, 422 (1968) ("In its original form, 42 U.S.C. § 1982 was part of the Civil Rights Act of 1866."); Saint Francis Coil. v. Al-Khazraji, 481 U.S. 604,612 (1987) (stating that § 1981 has its roots in both the Civil Rights Act of 1866 and the Voting Rights Act of 1870).
6. Singer v. Denver Sch. Dist. No. 1,959 F Supp. 1325, 1327–28 (D. Colo. 1997).

Petit-mal Seizure

42

Patrick Wright

It is far from normal how Patrick's life started in a garbage can and settled in as the Director of Trauma Anesthesia at Trinity Hospital. After 40 years of anesthesia practice, he announced that he would be retiring at the end of the year. He was legendary in the role of teacher and clinician. He had this "thing" where he would talk out loud what was going on in his brain when evaluating a complex case. It was a talent to hear the extreme confidence bounce off his self-doubt. He only did this in the hospital, but his wife would differ.

Patrick's whole body and soul were literally outside the box. On the second day of his life, he was found on the steps of the Metropolitan Museum of Art in New York City. There was an anonymous note that was profoundly sad and from his mother. She had no resources to raise Patrick.

Patrick was examined by a pediatrician and blood was sent for genetics with the usual CBC and metabolic panel. A CT scan of the head was completed. The fontanelles were normal.

Carolyn and George Martin were beaming on the drive home with their adopted baby, Patrick. He grew up with parents who were wealthy. From pre-K through the eighth grade, Patrick attended the Academy of the Sacred Heart. His high school years were at Deerfield Academy in Deerfield Massachusetts. Patrick was a B+ student and did not have the grades for the elite colleges in Massachusetts. He was accepted with pride, to Rice in Houston Texas. His GPA from Rice was 3.4. His SAT score defined mediocrity. His father wrote a check that was sufficient for most medical schools. Trinity accepted the "bribe" and accepted him. Patrick chose anesthesia as his field of medicine. He became an expert in surgical intensive care, starting with his Critical Care fellowship and a 5-year experience as a faculty member at Emory. Patrick married his office mate at Emory. Nancy Russo who was from New Orleans and Patrick knew that he would be moving to New Orleans just minutes after he put his wedding ring on Nancy.

A 62-year-old male, presented for an open eight-centimeter abdominal aortic aneurysm repair. His complex medical history included hypertension, two stented

C. Scher, *Anesthesia Conversations*,
https://doi.org/10.1007/978-3-032-05354-1_42

coronary artery diseases, atrial fibrillation, adult-onset diabetes, COPD, glaucoma, and peripheral vascular disease. While he no longer smoked, he quit his two-pack-a-day habit at age 40.

With his comorbidities, essential evaluations and treatments had to be addressed before the repair of his aneurysm:

1. A CT PET scan is a nuclear study to assess the coronary artery perfusion of the myocardium
2. Duplex ultrasound of the carotid arteries to determine plaque in the carotid arteries.
3. Blood for a metabolic panel, including liver function and kidney function
4. CBC, type, and cross
5. PT-PTT
6. Frailty scoring
7. Baseline cognitive function test

The original plan was an endovascular aortic repair. However, imaging revealed a tortuous aorta with multiple areas of calcification. The iliac vessels were too small in diameter to open to accommodate instrumentation for aortic stent placement. An open "triple A" (abdominal aortic aneurysm) was the operation of choice.

Patrick had not seen an AAA done in years. He chose to do that case since he would be the physician in charge of his critical care. Patrick had a resident who suggested:

1. Thoracic epidural for postoperative pain management
2. Awake arterial line
3. A two-stick right internal jugular catheterization. One wire for a triple-lumen catheter and the second wire for an introducer/pulmonary artery catheter
4. Lumbar drain

Patrick agreed and disagreed at the same time.

"Other than the thoracic epidural, why torture the man by doing all of these procedures awake. If he had significant coronary artery disease, an awake arterial line is overrated."

A lumbar drain was placed to maintain perfusion of the spinal cord. CSF is drained to protect the perfusion of the spinal cord

The induction and maintenance of anesthetic were uneventful. Two units of PRBCs were administered. Urine output exceeded 100cc every hour. CSF did not need to be removed.

While on skin, the surgical attendant made his way over where Patrick was sitting.

"Great job Patrick"

Patrick did not respond. He was just staring at the operating room bed. He was aphasic and did not grab the cup of coffee that was handed to him. The resident volunteered to get some orange juice: hypoglycemic?

Patrick was sent for a CT-angio of the brain. There was no evidence of a clot or subarachnoid bleed. The CBC was normal, but the metabolic panel revealed a mild metabolic acidosis and a lactate of 4. The echocardiogram was normal except for images of the right ventricle. The right heart looked empty. The urinalysis had a very high specific gravity. The ABG had hematocrit of 50 and platelet count of 500K. The WBC count was normal with a normal distribution of lymphocytes and granulocytes.

A physical examination that was consistent with profound dehydration with a high fragility score consistent with protein-calorie malnutrition. Patrick was admitted to the medical intensive care unit. The working diagnosis was severe dehydration, exhaustion, and starvation. An intravenous was placed, and 2 liters of Lactated Ringers were administered.

Psychiatry was called to make an assessment. Two psychiatrists agreed that this episode was a panic attack. If Patrick were awake and alert, he would think that the diagnosis of a panic attack was ridiculous.

Patrick's anesthesia resident lost it. "All of the testing resulted in only one possible conclusion. Patrick was dehydrated at its worst. You do not have a lactate of 4 from a panic attack, for fucks sake."

Patrick's staring and aphasia started before there were any signs of a panic attack. The signs and symptoms of a panic disorder include chest pain, palpitations, dyspnea, sweating, nausea, the sensation of choking, chills, and feelings of depersonalization. Patrick did not have any of them. His "Spell" lasted five minutes.

Zoloft and Clozapine were prescribed, and he thought the assessment and management of a panic attack was inane. He never filled the scripts and did not attend the psychiatric clinic visit that was ordered.

Patrick wanted an assessment from a neurologist. He was concerned that the possibility of a seizure was not explored. Moishe Leventhal was a Professor of Neurology with a subspecialty in seizure disorders. Patrick's neurological exam was normal. Dr. Leventhal probed Patrick's history in detail. He had two episodes this year, both starting with lip smacking: one in a movie theatre with his wife present and a second episode in his office observed by his physician assistant. Those cases were so short-lived that they did not see a reason to mention them to anyone.

"Patrick, I believe you are having Petit-mal seizures that are also known as Absence seizures. It will show up on an EEG as an abnormality."

The EEG did find the focal point in his brain where the seizures emanated from. There was no confusion with respect to his diagnosis. Ethosuximide was prescribed as a first-line treatment of choice for Petit-mal seizures.

"If not treated, you cannot drive, take care of patients, and any activity that requires 100 % attention like swimming. The rules regarding driving differ from state to state. Let's start you on a perampanel. If you are seizure free for 12 months with medication, you can start driving after a year. If you work with residents or nurses who are aware of your seizure history, you can start with a month of perampanel under your belt. These regulations are mine and are conservative."

The guidelines suggested by Dr. Leventhal were painfully restrictive. Patrick did not want to put anyone in danger. He would follow Dr. Leventhal's guidelines; however, he would never drive again.

Suggested Reading

1. Asadi-Pooya AA, Zeraatpisheh Z, Barzegar Z, Jafari A, Hashemi E, Sadeghi A, Setayesh AS, Tahmasbi Z, Zahadatpour Z. Driving restrictions in patients with seizures; a review of the regulations from the English-speaking nations. Epilepsy Behav. 2022;135:108888. https://doi.org/10.1016/j.yebeh.2022.108888. Epub 2022 Sep 9.PMID: 36095874
2. Bandelow B, Allgulander C, Baldwin DS, Costa DLDC, Denys D, Dilbaz N, Domschke K, Eriksson E, Fineberg NA, Hättenschwiler J, Hollander E, Kaiya H, Karavaeva T, Kasper S, Katzman M, Kim YK, Inoue T, Lim L, Mandrakis V, Menchón JM, Miguel EC, Möller HJ, Nardi AE, Pallanti S, Perna G, Rujescu D, Starcevic V, Stein DJ, Tsai SJ, Van Ameringen M, Vasileva A, Wang Z, Zohar J. World Federation of Societies of Biological Psychiatry (WFSBP) guidelines for treatment of anxiety, obsessive-compulsive and posttraumatic stress disorders-Version 3. Part 1: anxiety disorder. J World J Biol Psychiatry. 2023;24(2):79–117. https://doi.org/10.1080/15622975.2022.2086295. Epub 2022 Jul 28.
3. Crunelli V, Lőrincz ML, McCafferty C, Lambert RC, Leresche N, Di Giovanni G, David F. Clinical and experimental insight into pathophysiology, comorbidity and therapy of absence seizures. Brain. 2020;143(8):2341–68. https://doi.org/10.1093/brain/awaa072.
4. Narayanan N, Selvaraj S, Mohamed Khalifa A, Gaur A, Kaliappan A, Reddy KS. Seizure in geriatric population – an unheeded integer. J Family Med Prim Care. 2023;12(4):644–8. https://doi.org/10.4103/jfmpc.jfmpc_1613_22. Epub 2023 Apr 17
5. Xu Y, Shanthosh J, Zhou Z, Somerville E, Anderson CS, Glozier N, Hackett M. Prevalence of driving and traffic accidents among people with seizures: a systematic review. Neuroepidemiology. 2019;53(1–2):1–12. https://doi.org/10.1159/000500599. Epub 20 May 24.PMID: 3112967

Creutzfeldt–Jakob Disease (CJD) 43

Travis Young

Travis Young was a regional anesthesia freak! If a block could be done, he would "market" it to his patients. His selling points to the patient included the elimination of PONV and analgesia for as long as the surgeon wanted with tunneled catheters. Ambulatory patients with regional anesthesia were discharged before those who received general anesthesia. The consumption of narcotics postoperatively was less in those who had blocks than in those without blocks.

Travis followed ASRA guidelines and was current with peer-reviewed papers on regional anesthesia. He was very conservative with patients on 10A inhibitors and drugs that had a negative effect on platelet function. He purchased a platelet function analyzer, not for the platelet count but for their function.

Travis's technical skills with ultrasound and his knowledge of the anatomy of the image on the screen, made him almost immune from trouble. He never needed more than two attempts. The cooperation of the patients was almost always excellent from his soothing manner mixed with his own concoction of medications. He gave out a cell phone number to patients and was meticulous with his follow-ups.

Travis lectured at the American Society of Anesthesiologists, The International Anesthesia Research Society, European Anesthesia Society, Karolinska, and ASRA. He won teacher of the year in his own department, University of Pennsylvania, five times despite his reputation of being egocentric, eccentric, ornery, and a ballbuster.

He respected his colleagues at Penn and wanted the residents to behave at the highest professional level. There were no jokes, and he made it clear that he was the only one on the planet who never cursed. He was intolerant of chatty conversation.

Over the years, he had been approached by companies that wanted to use Travis's name for their products, tailored for regional anesthesia. Travis wanted to design perfect products with safety, accuracy and precision. There was a sterilized kit for each nerve block. The price point was double the two competitive kits. To make the price cheaper, most of the items in a kit could be recycled, sterilized, and used again. The biomechanical division of the school ordered 50 recycled kits.

C. Scher, *Anesthesia Conversations*,
https://doi.org/10.1007/978-3-032-05354-1_43

Every "pre-used " item would be in a box with green print, as opposed to a new kit, where all of the contents were never used. The ultrasound device used was a Toshiba, and Travis recommended minor modifications; the device would shut down after 3 minutes if the probe was not covered with a sterile "condom."

Most of the components in "his" kit could be used five times. Batteries for nerve stimulation were tested after each use. At the end of the case, the box would be placed in a red carton for pick up. The price of each kit was 25% more, but it could in reality be used five times.

Anesthesiologists had a choice of the recycled kits or nonrecycled new ones. After a month, the breakdown was even. Those who used the new kit recorded a 50% reduction of "wet taps". It was unanimous that it was easier to see the new needle under ultrasound with the epidural needles that were designed by Travis. There were 25% less failed blocks. All of the paper in the kit was recyclable, including the box that held the contents. Over the course of a year, the use of Travis's designed kit was used in 80% of academic centers. Travis's name was on the front of every kit.

About one year after the introduction of Travis's recycled kit, there was a case report in JAMA of a patient who contracted Creutzfeldt–Jakob Disease (CJD). This neurocognitive disorder is a fatal degenerative brain disease. Memory loss, behavioral changes, movement disorders, hallucinations, myoclonus, and essentially all of the neurological problems that are seen with severe nerve degeneration. The case report was a neurosurgical case.

In total, 85% of cases of CJD occur for unknown reasons, while about 7.5% of cases are inherited in an autosomal dominant manner. Exposure to brain or spinal tissue to prions causes a cascade of events of misfolding of proteins that lead to a chain reaction where large clumps of proteins accumulate in the brain, causing neurodegeneration of the brain. There is no DNA or RNA in prions. The symptoms of CJD are caused by the progressive death of the brain's nerve cells.

The CJD prion is dangerous. It promotes refolding of the native prion protein into the diseased state. The number of misfolded protein molecules will increase exponentially, and the process leads to a large quantity of insoluble protein in affected cells.

There was no evidence that sporadic CJD could spread among people via normal contact or blood transfusions. An electroencephalogram, spinal tap, and magnetic resonance imaging supported the diagnosis.

There are only supportive treatments for patients with CJD: clonazepam, opioids, and anticonvulsant medications. The onset is around 60 years of age. The time from contact to clinical symptoms is not known. Once symptoms appear, death is certain within a year. The symptoms of CJD are caused by the progressive death of the brain's nerve cells.

People may develop CJD, if they carry a mutation that codes for the prion protein. This occurs in only 5–10% of all CJD cases. In sporadic cases, the misfolding of the prion protein is a process that is hypothesized to occur as a result of the effects of aging on cellular machinery, explaining why the disease often appears later in life. The majority of the diseases are sporadic, but in 5%, of the cases the disease is iatrogenic. Prions may not be inactivated by of routine sterilization procedures. The World Health Organization and the US Centers for Disease Control and Prevention recommend that instrumentation used in such cases be immediately destroyed after use.

Two years ago, there was a case report in a patient with CJD) from Seattle. The case was diagnosed by a medical student who had been reading her pathology book. The rapid and horrific clinical decline, along with MRI, EEG, and CSF analysis, led to the diagnosis. The investigation determined that a patient in an OR 10 underwent a craniotomy for a benign meningioma. He was discharged after two nights in the hospital. On postoperative day 8, there was a sustained change in behavior, myoclonus, dementia, movement disorders, and hallucinations. Supportive care was provided, and the patient survived for 15 months from the day of diagnosis.

JAMA published this patient with CJD as a case report. It has been read by thousands of physicians in most fields of medicine. Two years after the introduction of CJD, there was a second case report that read like the first. There was no neurosurgery involved, which muddled the diagnosis. The only procedure in this patient's life that could possibly be related to neural tissue was a labor epidural that ended with a "wet tap" by an anesthesia resident.

There were multiple attempts with this epidural, leaving several small holes in the skin with both blood and CSF dripping out. Due to the mess that the resident created, Travis took over and called for another epidural kit. Both kits used were from recycled boxes. The epidural seemed to speed up the labor process. Six months after the patient delivered, the horrific signs and symptoms of CJD declared itself. The patient survived for ten months after the diagnosis and died in hospice care.

The investigation of the "infection" was comprehensive, ranging from West Nile Virus to CJD. The clinical picture of the patient was the result of prions on the "sterilized" epidural needle that entered the CSF. The usual sterilization technique did not eliminate the prions on Travis's kit with the recycled epidural needles.

Travis went to the CDC website and saw the "cocktail" to sterilize prion-contaminated needles. Surgical instruments contaminated with prions can be sterilized by autoclaving using hydrogen peroxide gas. Travis had never heard of the word "prion."

He was advised not to make any attempt to sterilize the kits. The recommendation was simply to throw the kits out. Travis pleaded his case that throwing the kits out was a failed business strategy.

Travis tried to outsource the sterilization and recycling of the kits to a private company. The overwhelming consensus was that the recycled needles were the problem caused by the "wet tap." The root cause analysis determined that while there was a CDC recommendation for sterilization of prions, "why go there"?

Travis refused to take the blame. The mounting momentum boxed Travis out. He ultimately took the blame. The case made him: less arrogant, less ornery, less intolerant, but a better teacher and a critical listener. Most of the practicing anesthesiologists did not believe that the wet tap was the problem. Simply stated, it was just his day to "step in shit."

Travis knew that he needed to disappear. Any change would put him under the radar, a place that he never went to. Trinity needed his skills. Chris agreed that Travis "stepped in shit," but his ego drove him to develop his own kits. Travis looked at the map of the United States and put his finger on New Orleans. He had never been there yet; it was far enough from Penn. Chris made him an offer he had to take: a job.

Suggested Reading

1. Casey C, Sleator RD. Prions: structure, function, evolution, and disease. Arch Microbiol. 2024;207(1):1. https://doi.org/10.1007/s00203-024-04200-3. PMID: 39572454
2. Cazzaniga FA, Bistaffa E, De Luca CMG, Bufano G, Indaco A, Giaccone G, Moda F. Sporadic Creutzfeldt–Jakob disease: Real-Time Quaking Induced Conversion (RT-QuIC) assay represents a major diagnostic advance. Eur J Histochem. 2021;65(s1):3298. https://doi.org/10.4081/ejh.2021.3298.
3. Hervé RC, Hedges J, Keevil CW. Improved surveillance of surgical instruments reprocessing following the variant Creutzfeldt–Jakob disease crisis in England: findings from a three-year survey. J Hosp Infect. 2021;110:15–25. https://doi.org/10.1016/j.jhin.2021.01.005. Epub 2021 Jan 19.PMID: 3348229.
4. Kobayashi A, Kitamoto T. Mizusawa H.Iatrogenic Creutzfeldt–Jakob disease. Handb Clin Neurol. 2018;153:207–18. https://doi.org/10.1016/B978-0-444-63945-5.00012-X. PMID: 2988713
5. Uttley L, Carroll C, Wong R, Hilton DA, Stevenson M. Creutzfeldt–Jakob disease: a systematic review of global incidence, prevalence, infectivity, and incubation. Lancet Infect Dis. 2020;20(1):e2–e10. https://doi.org/10.1016/S1473-3099(19)30615-2. PMID: 31876504
6. Vacca VM. CJD: Understanding Creutzfeldt–Jakob disease. J Nurs. 2016;46(3):36–42; quiz 42-3. https://doi.org/10.1097/01.NURSE.0000480598.84274.0f. PMID: 26840797

Spinal Anesthesia Is Awful! 44

Thomas Bosa

Thomas Bosa wanted to become a journalist, and his twin brother Carlos wanted to follow their parents to the financial world. The big squeeze was on. Their dominating father made sure that they were in either a medical school or a law school. Thomas was accepted to the Emory University School of Medicine, and Carlos was accepted to the Emory University School of Law. No loans were needed for education. Their parents were wealthy. They lived on Audubon Place, a gated street for the super-rich in New Orleans.

Thomas remained at Emory for his anesthesia residency and a Master's in Public Health Policy. From the first day of his residency, Thomas put himself on a turbo-charged climb to become a Chair of a Department of Anesthesiology. He did not accept any teachings from a faculty member that did not include some evidence in "standard of care." He periodically poured over peer-reviewed clinical trials, ASA guidelines, and well-respected textbooks, such as Clinical Anesthesia, edited by Paul Barash. He would ruminate when told "you cannot do regional to a person under general anesthesia, or the cricoid pressure bullshit, the awake arterial line crap and the selling of the spinal anesthetic."

Everyone knew that Thomas and Carlos believed that so much of life was based on ignorance and lack of evidence. "There is a god? You must be kidding me, Spinal Anesthesia!! Do you really think patients like that experience? The patient has to be awake for a nerve block? What is the big fucking deal if I give succinylcholine, to a bed bound patient? Has anyone ever seen succinylcholine causing hyperkalemia in a bed bound patient? The entire SICU has bed bound patients who need an RSI with a full stomach from bowel akinesia from narcotics. Are bariatric cases considered full stomachs?"

Thomas always challenged conventional teachings that propagated through the years based on nothing. There were times when he was told that he was wrong. That was never a consideration for him.

Gary Lewis was a 67-year-old cowboy in the classical sense, presented for left total knee arthroplasty. His past medical history included a biventricular pacemaker

C. Scher, *Anesthesia Conversations*,
https://doi.org/10.1007/978-3-032-05354-1_44

from a total heart block that was inserted 5 years ago. Over the course of time, his heart stopped beating and became 100% paced. His EF was 65%, and his echocardiogram was entirely normal. He does not have pulmonary hypertension. The lack of any electrical activity in his heart was not a concern to his cardiologist, but he could never "wrap it around his head." His fear was constant. On a good day, his fear was not zero, but was a 5. He zoomed to 10 with the smallest provocation.

Mr. Lewis had medically controlled diabetes on Metformin with blood levels of glucose ranging from 100 to 125. He had no signs of frailty, and his cognitive function was normal. He did not drink, smoke, or use any illicit drugs. He did not take any supplements. There was a questionable allergy to Bactrim.

His physical exam was unremarkable except for a visual scar from his pacemaker and right ACL. There were no limits on his physical activity. The remote interrogation of his pacemaker was always normal. Mr. Lewis swam four times a week, with each session lasting one hour. He is typed and crossed for two units. His CBC, basic metabolic panel, and clotting studies were all normal. It was standard to have his pacemaker reprogrammed for the case. The EP service was notified.

The anesthetic plan for knee arthroplasties was historically a spinal with sedation. The anesthetic was 2–4 mg of midazolam, a 12–15 mg hyperbaric spinal bupivacaine, and a propofol infusion for sedation. One gram of tranexamic acid was added to prevent fibrinolysis. Antibiotics were vancomycin and cefazolin.

The attending faculty asked a question that he knew would be answered with Thomas's bullshit. "Thomas, do you agree with the plan to proceed with a spinal anesthetic?"

"You know me. Of course I do not agree. I have read some papers that support general anesthesia over a spinal."

"You cannot make a statement or even an opinion without the name and year of the authors."

"Yes, sorry, I do not recall the names of the authors or project design. In the TKA cohort, subjects receiving GA had shorter time to reach discharge criteria, less dizziness and PONV, and better earlier ambulation compared with a spinal. Pain scores were lower after 6 hours with an opioid-sparing effect in the GA group compared with the spinal group. Patients in the GA group were more likely to favor the same type of anesthesia if they had to have surgery again. There were no significant differences in length of PACU stay, blood loss or complications between the two groups except urinary retention and a need for a Foley catheter was significantly higher in the spinal group."

"Thomas, you are not credible. You remember every detail of a paper, but you do not have the authors or the name of the journal. If I cannot cite my teaching, then I would not be credible but go on."

"It is difficult to believe that there was less PONV in the general cases. I have a bias against spinals in most cases except for C-sections." "You put a spinal in a senior patient, he buys a Foley for hours if not days. It takes time for the detrusor muscle to regain tone and strength.

Everything in these cases is about infection and a Foley is a danger to the new joint. Nurses are trained to use ultrasound of the bladder and make bladder rounds on those who have not peed. A straight catch is done when the bladder is full. The nurses usually have to straight cath a patient 2–3 times for the spinal patients. It is not uncommon for a senior patient to have an enlarged prostate where urology must be called to pass a Foley.

When I have interviewed patients who have had spinals, most say that they would not choose a spinal ever again!"

"For a student of facts, there are plenty of pieces of the puzzle of a spinal anesthetic that are not factual. There are so many confounding variables when you compare different anesthetics, Getting enough patients in a cohort when comparing spinals to general anesthesia virtually impossible."

Thomas's temper was ready to launch off. They talked about blood loss. "There are surgeons who finish a case in an hour and are 100% different from those who take 3 hours. The hematocrit that presses the button to transfuse is also so different among the surgeons and anesthesiologists. I only give blood products when there is no dispute about it. The surgeons want the patients to walk on day one. It is ridiculous. What is the point? The patients are miserable. This is a metric that needs not to be a metric."

The attending exasperation level started to climb and changed subjects. "Thomas, I see that you never use the BIS monitor."

"I was taught it was an awareness monitor. With a score less than 60, they remotely could be aware during a generic general anesthetic. scores. This is an example of not using a BIS in every case. It would be incredible if there was a dose response curve for anesthetics and BIS scores but there are none. Dosing anesthetics based on vital signs is problematic when patients are on beta blockers, antihypertensives and those with pacemakers. I have never seen or have heard of a case of awareness.

There is a research race to determine if general anesthesia causes neurodegeneration in babies under the age of two. If you believe that, a BIS monitor might have the clinician titrate the anesthetic to a higher score to avoid apoptosis, deposition of beta amyloid protein and tau protein but of course that is ridiculous."

Thomas sounded professorial. The attending anesthesiologist was impressed but exhausted by Thomas's continuous rebuttals. Thomas entered the "world of attending land," where the attendings were ready to pull the plug on him.

Thomas had the insight to determine that his relationships with his fellow residents and just about all the attendings were deteriorating. Thomas was not clear on the dynamics that he created. The Program Director and Chairman of the Department had a private meeting with the leadership attendings in the department. They wanted Thomas to transfer. It was simply too painful to work with him.

Thomas was devastated but accepted the advice given by the leadership of the department. The Chair was well connected to the Chairs of many departments and arranged a transfer for Thomas to USC-Keck School of Medicine. Thomas did not want to go to California. He just wanted to go home to New Orleans.

Thomas was able to arrange, without any help, a spot at Trinity. He was told that he was disgraced by his co-residents and that he disgraced himself. He did not know why.

Thomas had to have the last word. That was who he was. Other than being a pain in the ass, he had done nothing to hurt a single patient, and he had the highest scores on the in-service exam. There was only documentation that he was an excellent resident. He was told by his law school brother to "lawyer up."

Rather than hire lawyers who were way above his pay grade, Thomas requested a meeting with Chris and Lily. Chris contacted Thomas's Program Director and Chair. Thomas was described as a "rebel" and arrogant. In summary, he was an excellent resident with an edge that was hard to deal with.

After the meeting with Thomas, Chris definitely wanted Thomas. Academic challenges? Perfect. Chris needed a solid organ transplant anesthesia attending. Chris agreed to take Thomas only if he did a fellowship in transplant anesthesia. Chris made a second criterion for accepting Thomas. Lily would be monitoring his "mood disorder." Chris was spot on with his perception.

Lily was not thrilled with Chris's decision. " Why are we taking him?" There is no upside here. I have never heard of an applicant who had terrible recommendations. All we were hearing was that Thomas was a pain in the ass. Gheeezus!"

Chris had great instincts. He was wrong with Thomas. Thomas tortured the Trinity faculty with a fervor that matched his time at Emory. Chris promised Thomas a position after he completed his solid organ transplant fellowship, and Chris could not break that promise.

Suggested Reading

1. Birenbaum A, Hajage D, Roche S, Ntouba A, Eurin M, Cuvillon P, Rohn A, Compere V, Benhamou D, Biais M, Menut R, Benachi S, Lenfant F, Riou B, IRIS Investigators Group. Effect of cricoid pressure compared with a sham procedure in the rapid sequence induction of anesthesia: The IRIS Randomized Clinical Trial. JAMA Surg. 2019;154(1):9–17. https://doi.org/10.1001/jamasurg.2018.3577. PMID: 30347104
2. Brueske B, Sidhu MS, Schulman-Marcus J, Kashani KB, Barsness GW, Jentzer JC. Hyperkalemia is associated with increased mortality among unselected cardiac intensive care unit patients. J Am Heart Assoc. 2019;8(7):e011814. https://doi.org/10.1161/JAHA.118.011814. PMID: 30922150
3. Ramirez MF, Gan TJ. Total intravenous anesthesia versus inhalation anesthesia: how do outcomes compare? Curr Opin Anaesthesiol. 2023;36(4):399–406. https://doi.org/10.1097/ACO.0000000000001274. Epub 2023 Jun 19.PMID: 37338939.
4. Stewart J, Gasanova I, Joshi GP. Spinal anesthesia for ambulatory surgery: current controversies and concerns. Curr Opin Anaesthesiol. 2020;33(6):746–52. https://doi.org/10.1097/ACO.0000000000000924. PMID: 33002959

Ultrasound-Guided Nerve Block: Intralipid Failure

45

Hesh Green

Hesh Green was a soft-spoken, kind, and compassionate anesthesiologist. Most resident training centers have a single attending assigned to a new resident for the first month of the academic year. The faculty who was assigned to him was a teacher of the year countless times and was known as being patient and a true advocate for residents.

Hesh did his work, went home, and then returned every day. He needed to be in a Shomer Shabbos residency: a program that allowed him to participate in the rituals that go with being an Orthodox Jew. He could not work on the Sabbath: Friday and Saturdays. He had to be off for all Jewish holidays. He arrived early every day so that he could have a private place and wrap himself with Tefillin, a set of small black leather boxes with leather straps containing scrolls inscribed with verses from the Torah. This ritual was for men only. The smoldering resentment started with his classmates for the special treatment he needed.

Hesh knew next to nothing when he started his anesthesia residency. Most residents have already had a rotation of two months in anesthesia during their third or fourth year in medical school. Hesh Green did not.

Unlike his coresidents in his class, he had not succeeded at a single intubation or intravenous placement during his first month of training in his anesthesia residency. His first month attending had never seen this before.

There was not a sympathetic coresident. All of the residents had learned the basic skills of endotracheal intubation and intravenous placement. While on call, Hesh could not be left alone. An additional resident had to take a call just to cover him. His confidence was completely broken.

Lily volunteered to help Hesh. She assigned herself to Hesh. She believed that she could get him on the path, but after one week, she thought he should resign. Anesthesia was not the field of medicine for him. Chris replaced Lily. He, unlike the others who tried to help Hesh, got it done.

In the first week of October, Hesh started to become successful with intubations and IVs. While having the highest scores on all examinations, He never caught up

C. Scher, *Anesthesia Conversations*,
https://doi.org/10.1007/978-3-032-05354-1_45

clinically with his classmates. By mid-year, her procedural skills were barely adequate. He kept it under wraps, the growing fear of hurting a patient. He would ask for help in every case.

Lily and her co-faculty members thought that he would never function as a provider in an operating room. With one year left, Hesh saved himself.

Hesh found his calling with his skills in regional anesthesia. His regional skills were at the top of his class. His classmates finally dropped their bias against his special treatment. Somehow, he became a respected asset to the program. His compassion for care, humanism, and even sense of humor came out. His peripheral nerve blocks were now seamless but needed a CRNA to do the rest of the case for the next step of clinical management. Every faculty member was surprised that Chris added Hesh to the faculty. With his interest in research, regional anesthesia, and teaching, Chris found value.

A 25-year-old male, with a history of heroin abuse, fell down a flight of stairs and sustained a fracture of his radius and ulna. He was on 50 mg of methadone, and his compliance with recovery was unclear. An infraclavicular block was strongly recommended for postoperative pain management in this addict. Three or four days with narcotics would be a failure.

The patient received 25 mg of intravenous methadone which is half of the PO dose. There were no cardiac cases that day. The cardiac attending anesthesiologist was assigned to the "block room." A senior resident, who had a comprehensive rotation in regional anesthesia a few months back, could do the block "in his sleep" and took control. The block was done with ultrasound guidance.

A total of 10 ml of 0.5% bupivacaine with 10 ml of 2% lidocaine was injected. There were no signs of an intravascular injection. Twenty minutes after the block was placed, it was easily assessed that the block did not work. Hesh was called to help. There were several questions that Hesh asked as he investigated the previous block. Hesh wanted to dissect and teach each component of a block to ensure success.

"The choice of the ultrasound probe used could give an image that does not define the exact anatomy that you are looking for. Frequency refers to compression on the skin and rarefactions in a sound wave. A higher frequency results in better resolution but limited penetration. Because the target is superficial, it is best to choose a higher frequency for superficial structures, while a lower frequency for deeper structures Attenuation is a property of ultrasound when it travels through tissues. A longer distance of travel and higher frequency waves result in greater attenuation. The alternative, the curvilinear probe will work, but the skill required has to be taught.

Where did you look to find the cords that needed to be blocked? The landmarks are the midpoint of a line from the middle of the jugular notch and the ventral process of the acromion which translates to just medial to the coracoid process, inferior to the clavicle. The goal being local anesthetic spread around the axillary artery. This is at the cord level of the brachial plexus.

Another approach being transducer position approximately parasagittal, just medial to the coracoid process and inferior to the clavicle. The arm is extended beyond the head and bent at the level to view the vein. If you cannot find the vein but are sure that you are seeing the artery, do not fret. Just keep proceeding with the block.

The needle should be a 22 gauge, 8–10 cm or a Tuohy needle if you are going to tunnel a catheter. If you do not see the needle, make sure the needle is under the shower of the ultrasound. The vein, artery and nerve are tightly packed together so nerve sparing is less likely.

Common effects include phrenic nerve block leading to some level of respiratory distress. A young healthy patient will do well with this block. Those that do poorly if the phrenic nerve is included are patients with COPD, or other lung disease that is impacted by the hemi-diaphragm. Horner's Syndrome is always a distinct possibility.

There are two ways of injection. 1. A single injection must impact the posterior cords. 2. Inject each nerve, one at a time. Make sure the posterior cord is injected. Hydro-dissection is essential. The choice of local was 10 cc of 0.5 bupivacaine and 10 cc of 2% Lidocaine. The lidocaine will quickly tell you if the blocking. Other choices of local anesthetic may be used as long as one is short acting and the other is long acting."

Hesh decided to redo the block. They put this patient on hold and did a two-hour case instead. Hesh watched his senior resident with the block. Visualization of the artery, vein, and nerves was crystal clear. Hesh told the resident to inject to view hydro-dissection. Hesh was satisfied and asked the patient if his arm was getting heavy. There was no response by the patient. Within seconds, the patient had a short grand mal seizure followed by cardiac asystole. Hesh was shocked. CPR was quickly started, and Hesh quickly intubated the patient.

A bolus of 2 mg/kg of intralipid was "pushed," and an infusion of 2 ml/kg/hour was started. There was no response to the bolus. CPR never stopped. Hesh screamed out to run an ACLS code with drugs. Hesh arranged for STAT cardiopulmonary bypass.

A second bolus of intralipid was given with no effect. Intralipid may not work if it is expired or has been frozen. There was no response to epinephrine. After 10 min of CPR, the patient was on bypass.

After an hour of cold bypass, the patient was warmed. A starling curve was generated with 100 cc of LR given sequentially. The heart started to beat, and by eyeballing the heart, it looked great. The pupils of the patient were equally responsive to light,

The patient did well without any neurological deficit. He was sent to the ICU and was discharged after 2 days. Hesh had to have the last word.

"For those of you that think that I am no longer frightened to work in an operating room, you are wrong. That fear is still here."

Suggested Reading

1. Abdallah FW, Macfarlane AJ, Brull ARE. The requisites of needle-tonerve proximity for ultrasound guided-regional anesthesia: a scoping review of the evidence. Reg Anesth Pain Med. 2016;41(2):221–8. https://doi.org/10.1097/AAP.0000000000000201. PMID: 25785841
2. Kamel I, Ahmed MF, Sethi A. Regional anesthesia for orthopedic procedures: what orthopedic surgeons need to know. World J Orthop. 2022;13(1):11–35. https://doi.org/10.5312/wjo.v13.i1.11. eCollection 2022 Jan 18. PMID: 35096534 Free PMC article. Review.
3. Kaye AD, Allampalli V, Fisher P, Kaye AJ, Tran A, Cornett EM, Imani F, Edinoff AN, Djalali Motlagh S, Urman RD. Supraclavicular vs. infraclavicular brachial plexus nerve blocks: clinical, pharmacological, and anatomical considerations. Anesth Pain Med. 2021;11(5):e120658. https://doi.org/10.5812/aapm.120658. eCollection 2021 Oct.
4. Muller SH, Diaz JH, Kaye AD. Clinical applications of intravenous lipid emulsion therapy. J Anesth. 2015;29(6):920–6. https://doi.org/10.1007/s00540-015-2036-6. Epub 2015 Jun 7

Anesthesia for a Complicated Cardiac Electrophysiologic Case

46

Anne Habid

A 68-year-old woman was transferred from a community hospital to Trinity with a diagnosis of total heart block that was treated with a dual-chamber pacemaker 1 year ago. She presented to the Trinity Emergency Department with the signs and symptoms of CHF. She was short of breath and required a 100% non-rebreathing face mask. Her vitals were a blood pressure of 70/40 with a paced heart rate of 100. Her temperature was 37.6, and her O_2 saturation before oxygen was 84. Her relative confusion improved with oxygen and her saturation improved to 94. Significant labs were elevated for BNP and Creatinine. BNP is a natriuretic peptide that is a biomarker for the severity of CHF.

An EKG suggested Pacemaker Syndrome. Pacemaker Syndrome is a combination of decreased cardiac output, loss of atrial contribution to ventricular filling, and loss of peripheral resistance response. When the timing between the two chambers goes out of synchronization, less blood is delivered on each beat. Her ejection fraction was 20%. The cure for her CHF was the removal of the dual-chamber pacemaker and the insertion of a biventricular pacemaker for re-synchronization of the right and left sides of the heart. The patient's daughter was fuming.

"Why did they not put a biventricular pacemaker in the first place! It is my understanding that CRT is never needed with a biventricular pacemaker. It does not matter if a lead cracks, the other lead is back up. Why was this not offered or at least discussed before the decision to implant a dual chamber pacemaker was made? Can I talk to the Chief of Cardiac Electrophysiology?"

The patient's daughter asked all the right questions. The daughter had done her homework after her dual-chamber pacemaker was placed. She never revealed that she was a physician.

Dr. Atticus Leo, the Chief of Cardiac Electrophysiology, was more than a procedure technician who was wealthy from his work. He was all about patient-centered care. He felt the humanism of "schmoozing" with his patients and family members. Dr. Leo chatted with patients about a wide array of subjects: " What is your favorite city? What do you like to do in your spare time? What are you going to eat when you

C. Scher, *Anesthesia Conversations*,
https://doi.org/10.1007/978-3-032-05354-1_46

get home?" Dr. Leo did not care about the answers. He wanted to be in the moment and earn trust. He is able to calm down the patient's daughter.

CHF in the ED consisted of Angiotensin receptor blockers and diuretics. By morning, she was comfortable at rest and consented to a biventricular pacemaker. Her case was scheduled for 1PM in the electrophysiology suite. The treatment for CHF was effective after 8 h in the Emergency Department.

Anne was concerned with the potential "hole in the heart" that could occur when the preexisting lead had to be removed. The EP electrophysiology cardiologist was not concerned. The lead was in the myocardium for only a year, and it should "pop right out. The protocol for all lead extractions stated that they all must be done in the main operating room and not in the suite."

The lead extraction must involve a cardiac surgeon and a bypass pump that is ready to go in case the extraction causes a hole in the heart. Anne felt strongly that the norm had to be followed. Anne checked with the blood bank; a type and screen had not been ordered. She needed to have the blood in the room before the case started. She thought the case should be done in the main operating rooms. If there was a problem, there were many anesthesiologists to help out.

Anne believed she was right. Anne had an undulating feeling about her career in anesthesiology. She had moments when she felt needed and effective, and all too often, disdain from the ded surgeons. She was a board-certified anesthesiologist, and there were too many times that her opinions were dismissed. Anne was the only physician in the room who did not want to proceed. It was time to get Chris involved.

Chris backed Anne 100%. Chris knew exactly what frustrated Anne. He instructed Anne to go with him to the cafeteria for coffee. They had cornered the EP team, and by the time they finished their coffee, Chris received a text that the case was ready to begin. There was a flurry of activity in the operating room as the bypass team was setting up. The massive transfusion protocol was available if needed and the case would be done in one of the main operating rooms. While relieved, Anne was pissed.

"Chris, what the fuck! What did you say to them."

"Exactly what you said, The main difference, and it is pathetic to say, but you are a woman. That comment stung them. It was so true. The last thing they wanted was a gender bias claim. I assured them I had 20 anesthesiologists ready to help them if need be. and that I would file a claim to the administration of gender bias. Simply, game over. There is one more item, they wanted the case done with only sedation. Anne, do you agree with that?"

" Of course not. The patient is very ill and sedating her to a point where she would not move would make her hypotensive. Now, they are making anesthesia decisions. Could you imagine us making electrophysiology decisions? Thank you Chris."

"Ok, you can intubate her, please do not give her sevoflurane. It suppresses any arrhythmias in the heart. I would like to map her. It is possible that an unknown tachyarrhythmia could play a significant role in this. She does have pacemaker syndrome but it is possible that her EF is so low from an electrical problem. The mapping takes about 25 minutes."

" I will do the case as a total intravenous anesthetic with a background infusion of norepinephrine.

Not that matters to you, my TIVA will be propofol, remifentanil and dexmedetomidine."

The induction of anesthesia proceeded without any difficulty. To keep the patient from moving. Anne kept the patient "deep." The norepinephrine helped to increase the depth of the TIVA. As they were securing the leads prior to making a pocket, the patient woke up! The dose of propofol was 150 mcg/kg/minute. Anne ran a checklist in her mind to explain the patient's wake-up. The infusion pump for propofol was fine.

"I have to turn on the sevoflurane. You are up to the pocket. Sevoflurane can no longer be the problem."

The EP team, as per custom, did not respond to Anne. The EP team started a new pocket.

" What the fuck, pus is pouring out of the pocket. Omg! What is going on here?"

Anne took a look.

"That is not pus! It is propofol! Somehow during the case, a vein from the intravenous propofol connected to a vein in the pocket. To be clear, the patient woke up because propofol was pouring into the vein and not into the brain."

"This is a contaminated case. We will not put the generator in a pocket. We will exteriorize the generator, start her on antibiotics for 7 days and put the generator into a new pocket. I know that this approach may be way to conservative, but we cannot take any chances with her."

The patient was discharged after three days and was converted to PO antibiotics. A clinic appointment was made 2 weeks later to determine the EF from synchronization with another ECHO. The clinic ECHO showed an EF of 40% and at the 4-month time period, the EF was 55% Anne followed the patient for those 6 months and felt great about her job.

Suggested Reading

1. Beck H, Curtis AB. Right ventricular versus biventricular pacing for heart failure and atrioventricular block. Curr Heart Fail Rep. 2016;13(5):230–6. https://doi.org/10.1007/s11897-016-0299-3. PMID: 2755389
2. Bontempi L, Vassanelli F, Cerini M, D'Aloia A, Vizzardi E, Gargaro A, Chiusso F, Mamedouv R, Lipari A, Curnis A. Predicting the difficulty of a lead extraction procedure: the LED index. J Cardiovasc Med (Hagerstown). 2014;15(8):668–73. https://doi.org/10.2459/JCM.0000000000000023.
3. Cao Z, Chen X, Su L. Hou X Cardiac resynchronization therapy for patients with heart failure and nonspecific intraventricular conduction delay. Pacing Clin Electrophysiol. 2023;46(8):913–23. https://doi.org/10.1111/pace.14791. Epub 2023 Jul 21.PMID: 37477568 Review
4. Guglin M, Barold SS. The role of biventricular pacing in the prevention and therapy of pacemaker-induced cardiomyopathy. Ann Noninvasive Electrocardiol. 2015;20(3):224–39. https://doi.org/10.1111/anec.12245. Epub 2015 Jan 6

47 Systolic Anterior Motion

Nina Anzalone

Nina spit out the Nicorette at the same time that she peeled the NicoDerm off her arm. With the locker opened, she opened up the carton of Marlboros. Her life had become unhinged, and this was not the time for abstinence. Nina pulled the filter off and smoked away. Her cigarettes had always been her Xanax, and she got herself together by the end of the second cigarette.

Nina had had to process the reality that her smokes no longer calmed her. She chose "cold turkey." During the anxious moments, she would wash her face, down a cold brew, and change her scrubs. Nina's yellow teeth were testimony to her abuse. Her addiction started 10 years ago when she was offered a cigarette during the second year of her residency. She did not believe at that time that her "smokes" would overpower her will.

Her resident texted her that they were ready to start the process of weaning the patient off bypass. Nina swished her mouth with Listerine and made her way back to the operating room.

Nina had a pedigree educational background: an undergraduate at the University of Washington, Medical School at the Mayo, and her Cardiothoracic Fellowship at Stanford. She flew up the academic ladder from Chief Resident to Assistant Professor, Associate Professor, and Full Professor in only 5 years after her fellowship. Her clinical expertise and published research were in transesophageal echocardiography and were very much appreciated by the cardiac surgeons. Nina had a national reputation from her activities in multiple committee chair positions of the ASA. And then, something very wrong was happening in her life.

It started a month ago. At the end of a hard day of work, Nina was unable to find her car in the Trinity Parking Garage. She always parked on the fourth floor by the stairwell. The car was not in the usual spot that she had been using for years. She went from the first floor to the fourth floor stairwell, and the car was "lost." Nina made her way to the Security Department and claimed that her car might have been stolen. Security combed the entire garage, and the car was not in the garage. A security officer drove Nina home, and her car was in her driveway.

C. Scher, *Anesthesia Conversations*,
https://doi.org/10.1007/978-3-032-05354-1_47

"Thank God, someone returned the car. How would they know where I lived?"

Nina did not drive to work. A colleague had driven her to work, and Nina did not remember that.

A week later, Nina arrived at work at 6AM. She never wore scrubs outside the hospital. There was always a clean pair of scrubs in her locker. She had a key lock. Nina turned the key, and the door remained locked. She made several attempts and then lost her temper. She kicked the locker door furiously until the locker no longer looked like a locker. Her locker was just outside the main door of the operating room. She was not even close to her locker—different floor, different wing.

The last event that led to her psychiatric and neurologic assessment was that she could not remember her cell phone number. She opened up her phone and went to the Department's Intranet. The names of all of the faculty members were listed alphabetically. She found all of her contact information, which included her cell phone. Nina started to cry and had her mother make an appointment for her with a neurologist. Nina took a leave of absence.

Dr. Boris Meuller was a psychiatrist whose specialty was memory loss related to substances in the environment. He was the third physician to evaluate Nina. It was conclusive that Nina needed an Amyloid PET Scan. She refused the scan. She did not want to know if she had early Alzheimer's. There is a strong link among senior family members of Alzheimer's disease. Nina was 43 and was fully aware of her family's history. Her father passed from early-onset Alzheimer's.

Dr. Meuller did an extensive history and performed the physical in the old-fashioned, and comprehensive way. Nina was a beautiful woman who counted every calorie she ingested. Breakfast was black coffee with two scrambled eggs, lunch was two cans of Bumblebee tuna, and dinner was pasta with pesto. She did not count the calories of the two martinis that she had every night.

The first word that Dr. Mueller spoke at the end of his exam was "BINGO"! He ordered a methylmercury level. The two cans of Tuna every day caused mercury poisoning. The blood test confirmed it. Dr. Mueller arranged for chelation therapy. Each treatment lasted 3 hours. The number of infusions depends on the mercury levels in the blood. After three 3-hour infusions, Nina was getting back to herself.

Nina's stat beeper went off for a case, two operating rooms away. Alan Klein, a superior surgical clinician, needed Nina for help.

The patient was a 45-year-old male with a past history of uncontrolled hypertension and type 2 diabetes mellitus who was in the intensive care unit with severe abdominal pain with guarding. An abdominal flat film revealed some possible air under the diaphragm, and arrangements were made to transfer the patient to the operating room for an abdominal laparoscopy or laparotomy. His ABG was significant for a mild metabolic acidosis and a lactate of 6. Only scant and concentrated urine was in the Foley. The blood pressure recorded was 70/40.

The ECG on the anesthesia monitor was alarming with a sinus tachycardia of 120 beats per minute. Nina dropped a TEE probe down the esophagus. She was initially unimpressed with the initial images; normal biventricular function, concentric hypertrophy possibly secondary to his uncontrolled hypertension, mild MR, mild TR with and grade I diastolic dysfunction. The volume of blood in the heart appeared to be normal. A CVP for drug administration and an arterial line were placed without incident. A nasogastric tube on suction yielded 50 ccs of bilious fluid.

A norepinephrine infusion and fluids were added to treat a blood pressure of 70/40. The patient seemed unresponsive to the fluid administration. The surgeons and Nina were on the same page as the patient became more unstable. Whenever Nina increased the dose of the noradrenaline, the blood pressure, counterintuitively, dropped.

The induction of anesthesia did not cause hypotension. Gas insufflation, as predicted by Nina, bottomed out his blood pressure of 54/32. Epinephrine was added, and the unstable patient became worse. Nina needed more views. Small bowel obstruction patients are usually not this "sick."

"Hey y'all. Think big picture here. We are missing something. I think the lactate of six sent us down the path of sepsis and possible dead bowel. We keep on increasing the dose of norepinephrine as if he had developed a tachyphylaxis. It is his heart!"

The suspected pathology was confirmed as small bowel obstruction, diagnosed only minutes after incision. Nina's new TE views now revealed a turbulence mosaic pattern on color doppler in the LVOT (left ventricular outflow tract). The ME LAX (Midesophageal long axis) view confirmed a dynamic LVOT obstruction. There was asymmetrical septal hypertrophy predisposing this patient to SAM (Systolic anterior motion of mitral valve), causing dynamic obstruction (higher velocity gradient) in the LVOT. If it were systolic anterior motion (SAM), the pressors would only increase the LVOT obstruction.

The patient denied any cardiac disease when interviewed. The likely coexistence of excessive doses of pressors, a systemic inflammatory response from sepsis, and hypovolemia brought out a more than significant left ventricular outflow obstruction.

Epinephrine was tapered, resulting in normal biventricular contractility and a decrease in hyperdynamic function. A vasopressin infusion was started to help wean the epinephrine. The left ventricular end diastolic area on the TEE guided fluid administration. Beta-blockers were titrated to get the rate and hyperdynamic state under control. The gradients and turbulence in LVOT disappeared and the MR looked trivial as before.

Nina was a complete physician who was the consummate professional, teacher, and owned patient-centered care. Her instincts and experience led her to surmise that this was a cardiac case. Her message to the surgeons was for their education. The decline of the patient with increasing pressors was due to Systolic Anterior Motion or SAM.

"SAM, a dynamic LVOT obstruction can occur in cardiac cases post suboptimal mitral valve repair in the setting of a hypertrophied ventricle. Hypovolemia, vasodilation and tachycardia worsen the situation. Who would have dared to introduce beta blockers, taper off inotropes in a patient with low pressures? This case does highlight the occurrence of SAM in a non-cardiac case."

Suggested Reading

1. Finsterwald C, Alberini CM. Stress and glucocorticoid receptor-dependent mechanisms in long-term memory: from adaptive responses to psychopathologies. Neurobiol Learn Mem. 2014;112:17–29. https://doi.org/10.1016/j.nlm.2013.09.017. Epub 2013 Oct 7. PMID: 24113652.
2. Guigui SA, Torres C, Escolar E, Mihos CG. Systolic anterior motion of the mitral valve in hypertrophic cardiomyopathy: a narrative review. J Thorac Dis. 2022;14(6):2309. Teresa A Mulaikal, MD, FASE, Vivek K Moitra, MD, MHA, FCCM.
3. Manabe S, Kasegawa H, Arai H, Takanashi S. Management of systolic anterior motion of the mitral valve: a mechanism-based approach. Gen Thorac Cardiovasc Surg. 2018;66(7):379–89. https://doi.org/10.1007/s11748-018-0915-0. Epub 2018 Apr 3.PMID: 29616461 Review
4. van Weteringen W, Sterke F, Vlot J, Wijnen RMH, Dankelman JA. Automated control for investigation of the insufflation-ventilation interaction in experimental laparoscopy. PLoS One. 2023;18(5):e0285108. https://doi.org/10.1371/journal.pone.0285108. eCollection 2023. PMID: 37146021.

48 Fundamentals of Placing a Double-Lumen Tube in the Correct Position

Chris Landry

A 68-year-old male diagnosed with right upper lobe lung cancer was on the operating room schedule for a right upper lobectomy. There was no evidence of metastatic lesions outside of the lung. His past medical history was significant for 1–2 packs of cigarettes for 40 plus years. Other than COPD, there were no other medical problems related to his current diagnosis. An anesthesia consult was ordered. Chris examined the patient and ordered pulmonary function studies and a DLCO (Diffusing Capacity of the Lungs).

The three-tier system, from a simple ABG to having a patient walk on a treadmill with a pulmonary artery catheter, has been replaced. The DLCO (Diffusing Capacity of the Lung for Carbon Monoxide) is based on the strong affinity of carbon monoxide for red blood cells. The test involves measuring the partial pressure difference between inspired and expired carbon monoxide. A low DLCO is significant in pulmonary interstitial thickening, a loss of vasculature as seen in COPD, or an increase in pulmonary artery pressures. A normal DLCO is greater than 75% predictive up to 140% Mild disease is 60%. Moderate disease is 40–60% predicted, and severe is less than 40%. These tests are predictive, if a patient can tolerate one lung anesthesia.

Surgery is essential to the treatment of his cancer, and cases are, at times, done in situations when the FEV1 is less than 60% predicted and the DLCO is just above severe.

The plan was to move forward even with a low FEV1 and DLCO. Chris made his resident come up with the anesthetic plan: size 37–39 left-sided double-lumen tube, an arterial line, central line, BIS sticker, and thoracic epidural. Chris wanted to use a total intravenous anesthetic. While he thought that inhalational anesthesia was not disruptive to hypoxic pulmonary vasoconstriction, he wanted no stone left unturned; remifentanil, propofol, and dexmedetomidine.

With high flow oxygen (60) liters running in the patient's nose, the patient was placed in the sitting position for the thoracic epidural. The patient received small

C. Scher, *Anesthesia Conversations*,
https://doi.org/10.1007/978-3-032-05354-1_48

doses of midazolam that stopped at 2 mg. The resident completed the epidural in 10 min. The induction involved only activation of the three infusions: remifentanil, propofol, and dexmedetomidine. Chris wanted the induction to go slowly to avoid hemodynamic changes. When the bispectral index (BIS) was 40, 100 mg of rocuronium was administered. After direct laryngoscopy, a loaded fiberoptic bronchoscope holding the double-lumen tube passed easily through the vocal cords. The fiberoptic bronchoscope was placed through the bronchial port and advanced past the carina and steered into the left mainstem bronchus.

The scope was then passed through the tracheal port, looking for the blue cuff in the left mainstem bronchus. Chris wanted the inflated blue cuff not visible. This was different from the usual teaching, where the blue cuff can be seen by the bronchoscope down the tracheal lumen. Chris, who was extremely experienced and a regular in the thoracic operating rooms, taught that when you move the patient from the supine to the lateral position, the cuff, at times, herniates out. After turning the patient lateral, the scope is advanced down the tracheal lumen. If the top of the blue cuff is seen, then all is well. If the cuff is not seen, the tube is pulled back to where the cuff is just visualized from the tracheal port. If it is pulled back too far, the bronchoscope is placed down the endobronchial lumen and pulled back to see the carina. Then the same steps as for initial placement are repeated.

When clamping the tracheal port, the right side should not move, and breath sounds are only auscultated on the left side. When the left bronchial port is clamped, breath sounds are auscultated only on the right side. With the proper placement of a double-lumen tube, the application of clamping and de-clamping maneuvers should not change oxygen saturation.

Clamping the tracheal port and opening its top allows air to escape from the operative lung. The lung will not move with ventilation and will become atelectatic. This will activate hypoxic vasoconstriction and send deoxygenated blood to the ventilated lower lung for oxygenation. If the patient does desaturate, and the endotracheal tube is in the correct position, then there are only two possibilities. 1. hypoxic vasoconstriction (HVC) is not working in the operative lung, or 2. hypoxic vasoconstriction is working in the lower ventilating lung. If the lower lung cannot accommodate the deoxygenated blood from the upper lung, it is possible that there is significant disease in the lower lung. Hypoxic vasoconstriction is activated in the lower lung.

There is an effective solution for desaturation. A Mapleson D or Bains circuit can be attached to the port of the operative lung, and oxygen flow can be adjusted to improve oxygenation without expanding the lung. This technique is simply giving CPAP to the upper lung. If that technique does not improve the blood saturation, PEEP can be applied to the lower lung. If those maneuvers are not helpful, you can PEEP the upper lung and CPAP the lower lung.

If there are no Mapleson D circuits available, a soft tip suction can be placed in the ETT and passed down the lumen of the operative side. Oxygen is attached to the catheter and dialed to a level that improves the saturation but does not inflate the lung.

If the double-lumen tube cannot be passed, the next step would be to extubate the patient and place a bronchial blocker. There are many bronchial blockers on the market. All work well, and the choice of the bronchial blocker is one that the anesthesiologist is most comfortable with.

Chris favored the Univent® tube. The Univent's all-in-one design consists of a single-lumen endotracheal tube, plus an attached lumen that accommodates the movable bronchial blocker. The blocker facilitates surgery by collapsing the upper lung, keeping blood and secretions from freely flowing to the healthy lung.

The fluid strategy was to administer no more than a liter. Pulse pressure variation of the arterial line is not accurate in the lateral position. The fluid administration needs to be tempered to prevent pulmonary edema. Since most of these cases are done with laparoscopy, a Foley catheter was not inserted. The plan was always to extubate if possible.

The resident gave a total of 10 cc of local anesthetic in the thoracic epidural. The patient was extubated, and a 100% non-rebreathing mask was weaned down to a simple nasal cannula. His pain control was acceptable, and Chris left the PACU with the feeling of mission accomplished without incident.

He lit up a cigarette in his office and was scolded by everyone who walked by his office. He continued to smoke. Chris did not put out any cigarettes until it was done. He had his own rules. Again, he took a challenging case and made it look easy. In his mind, he was the best anesthesiologist in the department. He could do whatever he wanted. He never boasted when he had done an excellent job, but loved to talk about his cases and his decision process.

Suggested Reading

1. Bergmann A, Schilling T. Intraoperative ventilation approaches to one-lung ventilation. Anasthesiol Intensivmed Notfallmed Schmerzther. 2021;56(5):329–41. https://doi.org/10.1055/a-1189-8031. Epub 2021 May 26.PMID: 34038972 Review
2. Cano PA, Mora LC, Enríquez I, Reis MS, Martínez E, Barturen F. One-lung ventilation with a bronchial blocker in thoracic patients. BMC Anesthesiol. 2023;23(1):398. https://doi.org/10.1186/s12871-023-02362-z. PMID: 38057754
3. Clayton-Smith A, Bennett K, Alston RP, Adams G, Brown G, Hawthorne T, Hu M, Sinclair A, Tan J. A comparison of the efficacy and adverse effects of double-lumen endobronchial tubes and bronchial blockers in thoracic surgery: A systematic review and a meta-analysis of randomized controlled trials. J Cardiothorac Vasc Anesth. 2015;29(4):955–66. https://doi.org/10.1053/j.jvca.
4. Douglass P. One lung ventilation. Br J Hosp Med (Lond). 2022;83(6):1–2. https://doi.org/10.12968/hmed.2021.0547. Epub 2022 Jun 10.PMID: 35787162
5. Li XF, Jin L, Yang JM, Luo QS, Liu HM, Yu HA. One-lung ventilation for thoracic surgery. Tumori J. 2017;103(6):495–503. https://doi.org/10.5301/tj.5000638. Epub 2017 Jun 7.PMID: 28604996 Review
6. Şentürk M, Slinger P, Cohen E. Intraoperative mechanical ventilation strategies for one-lung ventilation. Best Pract Res Clin Anaesthesiol. 2015;29(3):357–69. https://doi.org/10.1016/j.bpa.2015.08.001. Epub 2015 Aug 28.PMID: 26643100

Anesthesia for Burned Patient

49

Amelia Tauron

Life on the oil rigs that litter the Gulf of Mexico is fraught with significant dangers, with fire being the greatest threat. West Jefferson Medical Center has the largest burn center in Louisiana. Amelia Tauron transformed her life as a general anesthesiologist to become a well-known and highly regarded "burn doctor." If a worker was involved in a fire and is transported to the burn center, life is truly one day at a time.

Amelia's cell phone rings incessantly, and in most cases, Amelia received a report from a rig involving a worker with severe burns from an explosion on the rig. Most patients are in the highest imaginable pain. Eighty percent will be intubated in the first hour. A thorough assessment of the entire body is done in minutes. Once Amelia sees that nose hairs are singed, or voices that are muddled, there has been fire in or around their airway. There is a gradual rise toward respiratory failure.

Early intubation, before respiratory failure, is at the top of the treatment algorithm. When the call has been made, the ICU sets up in each bed, based on the report from the rig or helicopter. All fluids are warmed. The massive transfusion protocol is activated. In severe burns, blood is cauterized, and transfusion begins upon the arrival of the patient.

All of the burn slots in the Burn SICU are large to allow for full surgical procedures and laminar flow to decrease infection. Silver sulfadiazine, silver nitrate solution, and mafenide acetate are commonly used for local wound care. For more severe infections, systemic antibiotics may be administered, with a choice of flucloxacillin, co-amoxiclav, and gentamicin.

A general surgical set is opened every four hours, which is in alignment with the loss of sterility. The anesthesia machine is checked daily by the anesthesia team, and antibiotics are "locked and loaded." The anesthesia cart contains ketamine, fentanyl, propofol, rocuronium, and video laryngoscopes. A percutaneous trach set is opened for the surgeons. If venous access is a significant problem, intraosseous lines can easily be placed and serve as excellent large-bore IVs.

C. Scher, *Anesthesia Conversations*,
https://doi.org/10.1007/978-3-032-05354-1_49

Monitors remain a challenge. EKG leads have an alligator clip that holds an 18-gauge needle that is plugged into the patient. Depending on the extent of the burn, the goal of lines is to have an introducer in the internal jugular, as well as the double stick triple lumen. The hands are more frequently than not severely burned. The femoral arteries become the next choice for an arterial line. The pulse oximeter and a standard blood pressure cuff are usually problematic, requiring real ingenuity. An arterial line may involve a cut down.

The most difficult goal to accomplish is fluid resuscitation. Amelia uses the Parkland formula. The Parkland formula starts after transfusion metrics are obtained. A TEE is helpful for fluid resuscitation unless there is a mouth burn; it is a safe assumption that the esophagus is probably burned. "Just rely on Foley and ABG for now!"

In the early resuscitative phase, hypovolemia due to capillary permeability is the greatest challenge. Thermal injury causes the release of inflammatory markers at the site of injury and systemically (mostly histamine). The inflammatory markers increase the capillary permeability throughout the body and cause a fluid shift out of the intravascular compartment.

The state of shock includes a decreased cardiac output and increased systemic vascular resistance. Burn shock is a combination of distributive, cardiogenic, and hypovolemic shock. It is essential to replace the fluid in the intravascular compartment to preserve tissue perfusion of vital organs. There have been several clinicians who have developed algorithms for fluid resuscitation, all based on body surface area

The goals for fluid resuscitation are as follows: 1. urine output greater than 0.5 ml/kg per hour, 2. a base deficit less than 2, and 3. systolic blood pressure greater than 90 mm Hg and clinically with peripheral palpable pulses.

Burns with greater than 15% body surface area (BSA) in adults need resuscitation, calculated by the Rule of Nines. Estimation of body surface area burned is based on assigning percentages to different body areas.

The Rule of Nines:

The entire head is estimated as 9% (4.5% for anterior and posterior). The entire trunk is estimated at 36% and can be further broken down into 18% for anterior components and 18% for the back. The anterior aspect of the trunk can further be divided into the chest (9%) and abdomen (9%). The upper extremities total 18% and thus 9% for each upper extremity. Each upper extremity can be divided into anterior (4.5%) and posterior (4.5%). The lower extremities are estimated at 36%, 18% for each lower extremity. This can be further divided into 9% for the anterior and 9% for the posterior aspect. The groin is estimated at 1%. According to the American Burn Association's practice guidelines, patients with greater than 15% total body surface area (TBSA) and non-superficial burns should receive intravenous fluid resuscitation. Lines can be placed even through burned skin if other alternatives are not possible to avoid delays in resuscitation.

The Parkland formula uses the rule of 9s to calculate fluid resuscitation. The Parkland formula states that 2–4 ml of Ringer's Lactate per kilogram of weight per percentage of body surface area burned, with the first half given over the first 8 h and the remainder given over the next 16 h. The Parkland formula implies 4 mL/kg/

TBSA (3 mL/kg/TBSA in children) = total amount of crystalloid fluid during the first 24 h." 4cc × Body Weight (70 kg)× 15% burned = 4200cc. Half of the fluid is given in the first 8 h.

There are some exceptions to low urine output, where a burn patient has rhabdomyolysis from burns and/or acute renal failure. These patients require fluids of 1 ml/kg hour. In these cases, "more is not better," and the risk of fluid creep can be as life-threatening as the burn injury itself. For this reason, infusion rates should be recalculated hourly, and rates should not be increased by more than 20–25%.

Amelia mentioned the crystalloid /colloid debate. Which crystalloid or which colloid? This was Amelia's most important question. "Why has this controversy not been solved? Those who are in the crystalloid camp have been using the Parkland or other formulas with Lactated Ringers. It has been used for over 50 years and that testifies to its success. The huge complication is from the destruction of endothelial cells and LR seeping into the extravascular space, causing a significant edema. No matter which fluid is chosen, all can have fluid creep. Many burn patients receive far more resuscitation fluid than predicted by the Parkland formula. The phenomenon termed "fluid creep" may lead to compartment syndrome of the extremities or abdomen. These factors challenge the Parkland formula that has excluded colloid use, the impact of goal-directed resuscitation, and the overzealous, on-the-scene crystalloid resuscitation.

"There are two choices of colloid; fresh frozen plasma and albumin. They both remain intravascular significantly longer than LR. Ultimately, through capillary leaks they flow into the extravascular space. They carry with it plasma causing edema. Albumin is known for "clogging up" the renal glomeruli leading as well as the products of rhabdomyolysis seen in most burn patients.

Amelia was in the crystalloid camp. To compare efficacy between colloids and crystalloids, the patients compared must have the same amount of body surface area, weight, age, type of burn (thermal vs. electric), equal amount of full thickness burns, medical history, equal need for pressors, preexisting injuries from the burn, and countless other confounding variables to make one cohort for comparison. These factors explain why the controversy may not be clarified.

Debridement of devitalized burn tissue was done daily. There was significant blood loss with the debridement, and transfusions were needed at least twice a week. Bedside ketamine is used in most cases. The pulmonary service does a bronchoscopy to determine if the fire damaged the lungs. Stents are placed if there is any narrowing in the major airways in the lung and are deployed before respiratory distress develops. Pulmonologists assess lung injury and determine if a stent will be needed.

Amelia was in charge of setting up pain management protocols. A PCA requires "pressing a button." If the hands are burned, PCA will be practical. The "1–10 question does not work. It probably should be a 10–20 question. The simple and reliable is the nurse's judgment and the use of hydromorphone at increments of 0.2 mg as needed. For intubated patients, narcotics on pumps are ideal, as safety is not a concern.

Amelia rounds three times a day for each patient. The patient's condition changes rapidly, and the providers must keep up.

Suggested Reading

1. Duchin ER, Moore M, Carrougher GJ, Min EK, Gordon DB, Stewart BT, Sabel J, Jo-Nes A. Burn patients' pain experiences and perceptions. Burns. 2021;47(7):1627–34. https://doi.org/10.1016/j.burns.2021.01.010. Epub 2021 Feb 15.PMID: 33642121
2. Elsheikh R, Makram A. Multidrug-resistant organisms: the silent plight of burn patients. J Burn Care Res. 2024;45(4):877–86. https://doi.org/10.1093/jbcr/irae075. PMID: 38695094
3. Evers LH, Bhavsar D, Mailänder P. The biology of burn injury. Exp Dermatol. 2010;19(9):777–83. https://doi.org/10.1111/j.1600-0625.2010.01105.x. Epub 2010 Jul 14.PMID: 20629737
4. Kirkland KD, Gratton A, Mentzer C, Kubasiak JC, Yon JR. Inter-facility transfers for burn patients with concomitant traumatic injuries. Burns. 2023;49(6):1267–71. https://doi.org/10.1016/j.burns.2022.11.004. Epub 2022 Nov 19.PMID: 36813603
5. Romanowski KS, Carson J, Pape K, Bernal E, Sharar S, Wiechman S, Carter D, Liu YM, Nitzschke S, Bhalla P, Litt J, Przkora R, Friedman B, Popiak S, Jeng J, Ryan CM, Joe V. American Burn Association Guidelines in the Management of Acute Pain in the Adult Burn Patient: a review of the Literature, a Compilation of Expert Opinion, and next steps. J Burn Care Res. 2020;41(6):1152–64. https://doi.org/10.1093/jbcr/iraa120.

Raynaud's and Scleroderma

50

Anne Habid

During her second year at Bennington College in Vermont, Anne Habid had her first "attack" of Raynaud's Syndrome. It was a "textbook case" involving all four extremities with a blue tint to her skin. The small vessels in her hands and feet were vasoconstricted. She averaged two attacks each week and suffered in class with them. The cold winters in Vermont and stress precipitated her misery. She bought into the culture of the College and did not want to transfer. She was one of the few in her class that was leaning towards medical school. Her small liberal arts college had mandatory premed classes.

Although there was a Yale-trained rheumatologist in town, she wanted a university medical center for a consultation. The University of Vermont was two hours and 45 min away, and Brigham and Mass General were in Boston, three hours away. She made an appointment at Brigham and Women's Hospital. She had to wait 10 days.

The rheumatologist in Boston confirmed the diagnosis of Raynaud's Syndrome and prescribed: 1. Calcium channel blockers, 2. Magnesium, 3. Antioxidant vitamins, 4. Niacin, 5. Consumption of omega oils, 6. Spicy foods, and 7. A trial of Botox. While Raynaud's patients are never cured, the frequency and intensity of pain can be significantly reduced. Her life span would not be reduced.

Anne left the cold. Her transcript was excellent, and she applied to medical schools only in the South. There were small pockets of Muslim communities in some of the southern states, but only New Orleans stood out for her, to feel accepted. Orleans Parish is the one single community where acceptance is the rule. The city was blue and was surrounded by a red state.

Anne was accepted to five medical schools. On her list, Tulane University was the warmest. She made an appointment with Dr. Joe Broussard, the Chief of Rheumatology at Tulane, after her first night call during her internship year. Her Raynaud's were under control. She just wanted someone to follow her in case her Raynaud's took over her life again.

Anne started her CA-1 year at Trinity, and her health spiraled down after only three months into the program. Anne had thickening and stiffening of her hands

C. Scher, *Anesthesia Conversations*,
https://doi.org/10.1007/978-3-032-05354-1_50

from excessive collagen. Her heart rate was 35. She reported a wide range of gastrointestinal symptoms from heartburn to diarrhea. Dr. Broussard was heartbroken. Anne appeared to have systemic scleroderma, which would impact the quality of her life.

A CT of the abdomen and chest was negative for collagen deposition. An upper GI endoscopy and colonoscopy were normal. The hope was that she had morphea where only the skin and joints of the hands are impacted. The quality and lifespan of her life depended on cardiac involvement.

Dr. Kushner was an electrophysiological cardiologist at Tulane. Anne's echocardiogram and endomyocardial biopsy were normal. There was no pulmonary hypertension. On EKG, Anne was diagnosed as having a total heart block, which was verified by an EP mapping. She was added to the already full schedule of cases. Dr. Kushner made her his second case. A biventricular pacemaker was inserted.

Dr. Broussard put Anne on CAR-T Therapy. Anne's T-Cell cells were collected and modified to destroy B cells that create autoimmune antibodies. CAR-T stands for chimeric antigen receptors. CAR-T treatment stops or slows down the progression of scleroderma. Her hands would never be normal.

Anne's illness was more than she expected. With proper management, she would have a normal life expectancy. Her heart muscle, lungs, and gastrointestinal tract were not involved. Her pulmonary function tests and chest CT scan were normal.

Anne kept Lily and Chris apprised of her case. She would need physical therapy targeted at her hands. There needed to be a significant improvement if she wanted to be an anesthesiologist. Lily thought that two months off for PT should determine if she was moving in the right direction. PT included gentle hand stretches, joint mobilization, heat therapy, and all exercises that increase the range of motion. At the two-month metric, Anne was confident she could practice anesthesia. Lily assigned herself for a week to restore Anne's confidence and judge if she was up for the task. She was.

During her training, Anne developed hypertension, which is not uncommon in scleroderma. Her blood pressure was controlled with Losartan, and there was no significant advancement in her disease. She was accepted into the cardiac anesthesia fellowship at Trinity and joined the faculty of the Trinity Department of Anesthesia.

Anne's disease progressed to her lungs over time with pulmonary hypertension after four years on the faculty. The pulmonary hypertension team at Tulane became involved and started treatment. With constant surveillance and treatment, she responded to every block in her health.

Her success in her career helped pave the path in her personal life.

Suggested Reading

1. Pauling JD, Hughes M, Pope JE. Raynaud's phenomenon-an update on diagnosis, classification and management. Clin Rheumatol. 2019;38(12):3317–30. https://doi.org/10.1007/s10067-019-04745-5. Epub 2019 Aug 16.PMID: 31420815
2. Sirufo MM, Magnanimi LM, Ginaldi L, De Martinis M. Primary Raynaud's phenomenon, very early and early scleroderma tips for a timely diagnosis. Eur J Intern Med. 2022;98:111–2. https://doi.org/10.1016/j.ejim.2022.01.036. Epub 2022 Feb 1.PMID: 35120748

3. Rongioletti F, Ferreli C, Atzori L, Bottoni U, Soda G. Scleroderma with an update about clinico-pathological correlation. G Ital Dermatol Venereol. 2018;153(2):208–15. https://doi.org/10.23736/S0392-0488.18.05922-9. Epub 2018 Jan 24.PMID: 29368844
4. Moaveni D, Cohn J, Brodt J, Hoctor K, Ranasinghe. Scleroderma and pulmonary hypertension complicate two pregnancies: use of neuraxial anesthesia, general anesthesia, epoprostenol and a multidisciplinary approach for cesarean delivery. Int J Obstet Anesth. 2015;24(4):375–82. https://doi.org/10.1016/j.ijoa.2015.05.001. Epub 2015 May 8.PMID: 26119257
5. Davis MP, Gutgsell T, Gamier P. What is the difference between palliative care and hospice care? Cleve Clin J Med. 2015;82(9):569–71. https://doi.org/10.3949/ccjm.82a.14145. PMID: 26366952
6. Wang X, Wu X, Tan B, Zhu L, Zhang Y, Lin L, Xiao Y, Sun A, Wan X, Liu S, Liu Y, Ta N, Zhang H, Song J, Li T, Zhou L, Yin J, Ye L, Lu H, Hong J, Cheng H, Wang P, Li W, Chen J, Zhang J, Luo J, Huang M, Guo L, Pan X, Jin Y, Ye W, Dai L, Zhu J, Sun L, Zheng B, Li D, He Y, Liu M, Wu H, Du B, Xu H. Allogeneic CD19-targeted CAR-T therapy in patients with severe myositis and systemic sclerosis. Cell. 2024;187(18):4890–4904.e9. https://doi.org/10.1016/j.cell.2024.06.027. Epub 2024 Jul 15.PMID: 39013470 Clinical Trial

Anesthesia and the Heart Transplant

51

Leon Wagner

A 50-year-old male was diagnosed with ischemic cardiomyopathy and was wait-listed for a heart transplant. His medical history included hypertension, diabetes, percutaneous intervention of coronary arteries with four stents, and a CABG with mitral valve repair four years ago.

Chris poked his head into the operating room. He had never seen his newest hire work, teach, and communicate with the surgeons so well. He was pleased with his flexibility and professionalism. The transplant service at Trinity had a full clinical partnership with Tulane University Medical Center. Leon Wagner bounced. between Tulane and Trinity. The service averaged 20 transplants per year. Leon was not overwhelmed with his workload.

The pre-transplant right heart catheterization showed a relatively high PVR (pulmonary vascular resistance). A normal value for pulmonary vascular resistance using conventional units is 0.25 to 1.6 mmHg·min/l. Pulmonary vascular resistance may be also be represented in units of dynes/sec/cm-5. or Woods units with 3.0 being the upper level of normalcy. The patient's pulmonary vascular resistance was 3.67 Woods Units, which is clinically significant. A level of 5 wood units is severe pulmonary hypertension.

The echocardiogram revealed an ejection fraction of 10%. Clinically, the patient was short of breath in bed and was oxygen dependent. There were episodes of non-sustainable ventricular arrhythmias. An AICD was implanted. The combination of an extremely low EF and an elevated PVR added significant risk to a heart transplant.

The pulmonary hypertension team wrote the order for prostacyclins. Prostacyclin-like drugs regulate blood vessel function, clotting, and inflammation. They maintain tissue health throughout the body, including the lungs. They induce progressive vascular remodeling associated with pulmonary hypertension that leads to narrowed, thickened pulmonary blood vessels and abnormal hemodynamics. ECMO would be inevitable without this treatment. An AICD are bridges to transplant. The Impella is a percutaneously inserted ventricular assist device that takes blood out of the left ventricle and sends it to the aorta. It works by spinning in a closed casing.

C. Scher, *Anesthesia Conversations*,
https://doi.org/10.1007/978-3-032-05354-1_51

The optimal position of the Impella device was further confirmed by color Doppler transthoracic echocardiography. Despite comprehensive therapy, the patient required ECMO urgently before a heart was found.

The heart transplant team contacted UNOS (United Network Organ Sharing). A transplant was imminent. Leon always needed the most information possible concerning the heart that was accepted for transplant. The country is divided into 11 regions. Louisiana is in Region 3 along with Alabama, Arkansas, Mississippi, Georgia, Florida, and Puerto Rico. There are multiple criteria to match an organ to a patient in waiting.

If the organ was coming from a region other than 3, it is likely that the organ was accepted from a donor outside of the region. For Leon, warm ischemia time must be as short as possible. This time is usually calculated from the time the organ gets harvested to implantation. The organ is kept cool and bathed with a preservative, University of Wisconsin Solution. With a long ischemia time, reperfusion injury is likely to make the patient hemodynamically unstable when the heart is perfused. Leon always gave calcium and a few low-dose pushes of 10 mcg epinephrine at the time of reperfusion

The shortest ischemia times are from a brain-dead patient. The donor with the longest ischemia time is a Donation after Cardiac Death (DCD). A patient who is alive but requires total life support and has no chances of survival is a possible donor. The patient cannot be "awake. The family and physicians must agree that a transplant from a DCD donor is acceptable.

After transport to the operating room, any therapy that is perceived to be uncomfortable is removed from life support, including extubation. Shortly after extubation, the heart must stop quickly to avoid a prolonged warm ischemia time. Once the heart stops, the transplant team needs to wait 5 min in case the patient autoresuscitates; then the harvest begins. Over the years, many of the steps have changed to minimize warm ischemia time and dramatically bring up the number of organs for transplant.

A repeat right heart cath was repeated post-impella. The PVR escalated to 4 Woods Units, and the right ventricle needed support. Leon initiated milrinone at 0.5 mcg/kg/minute and nitric oxide at 40 parts/million. This treatment did not keep the patient off ECMO.

After two days of ECMO there was a donor. The heart was of a 17-year-old who was hit by a car while riding his bicycle without a helmet. The donor had a massive cerebral hemorrhage and met the criteria of being a brain-dead donor.

The transplant was uneventful until it was time to wean the patient from CPB. The contractility of the RV, as seen on TEE and by simply eyeballing, it was suboptimal. The RV was dilated with the septum impinging on the left ventricular outflow tract.

A peripheral ECMO was preferred (to allow chest closure and prevent another re-exploration for decannulation) with a drainage into the right femoral vein. The correct position was confirmed by TEE. This position ensured adequate venous drainage.

Cardiac output monitoring was done via echo (TTE/TEE). There was a significant improvement by 48 h of ECMO. ECMO right ventricular flows were titrated to allow a successful weaning. The success of weaning was based on Leon's TTE/TEE skills. RV support was continued medically in the form of nitric oxide, epinephrine, and milrinone. There was a discussion concerning the placement of a right ventricular assist device, but there was enough improvement to just watch and wait.

Suggested Reading

1. Awad MA, Shah A, Griffith BP. Current status and outcomes in heart transplantation: a narrative review. Rev Cardiovasc Med. 2022;23(1):11. https://doi.org/10.31083/j.rcm2301011. PMID: 35092203
2. Abdul Hameed Andrew J. Swift·Samer Alabed David G. Kiely Athanasios Charalampopoulos., Assessment of right ventricular function—a state of the art. Curr Heart Fail Rep (2023) 20:194–207
3. Sathianathan S, Bhat G. Heart transplant donor selection guidelines: review and recommendations. Curr Cardiol Rep. 2022;24(2):119–30. https://doi.org/10.1007/s11886-021-01631-y. Epub 2022 Feb 18.PMID: 35179716
4. Tan Z, Roscoe A, Rubino A. Transesophageal echocardiography in heart and lung transplantation. J Cardiothorac Vasc Anesth. 2019;33(6):1548–58. https://doi.org/10.1053/j.jvca.2019.01.005. Epub 2019 Jan 7.PMID: 30709594
5. Truby LK, Takeda K, Farr M, Beck J, Yuzefpolskaya M, Colombo PC, Topkara VK, Mancini D, Naka Y, Takayama H. Incidence and impact of on-cardiopulmonary bypass vasoplegia during heart transplantation. ASAIO J. 2018;64(1):43–51. https://doi.org/10.1097/MAT.0000000000000623. PMID: 28777136
6. Vuthoori R, Heaney C, Lima B, Knisel A, Miller E, Kennedy K. Assessment of cardiac recovery in patients supported with venoarterial extracorporeal membrane oxygenation. ESC Heart Fail. 2022;9(4):2272–8.

The Aging Anesthesiologist

52

Lenny Boggs

Lenny Boggs practiced academic anesthesia for 40 years. He was an old-school academic with excellent skills needed for regional, obstetrical, and adult cardiothoracic anesthesia. At 70, he removed himself from cardiac anesthesia cases as his echo skills were declining. His clinical knowledge was comprehensive, and he served as an examiner for the ABA oral boards. He edited and wrote over ten textbooks and accumulated 50 peer-reviewed publications. Lenny was the teacher of the year 21 times, and his passion for the field had not waned. He was determined to work as long as possible. Mentoring students, residents, and junior faculty made him a legend. He left the Trinity Department of Anesthesia in the days that followed Hurricane Katrina and returned to the department 6 months after the department was back in business.

Lenny was blessed with three children who grew to be physicians. Two sons were surgical oncologists, and his daughter was a pediatric oncologist. Lenny's wife kept the ship afloat as a wife, mother, and an accomplished academic nephrologist. Time caught up to Lenny as he was now facing his first surgery for colorectal cancer. As far as advanced imaging and colonoscopy could tell, there was no evidence of metastatic disease. The proposed operation was a partial colectomy, diverting ileostomy, and prostate biopsy for his rising PSA compared to his last PSA.

At 70, Lenny knew too much. His main concern was his 70-year-old brain. Would there be lasting effects of general anesthetics on his brain? He had read some of the literature on neurotoxicity, neuroprotection, and cognitive impairment. Would he lose some academic edge from long-lasting anesthetics and the systemic inflammatory response from the surgery?

Lenny did not want to discuss the onset of some memory loss over the last two years. Was it from being old, or the beginning of a form of dementia? One day, he could tell a listener about the starting players on the New York Mets, and other days, he would struggle with the same question. He chalked it up to simply aging.

It was once thought that the brain would return to its preoperative state, but science is clear that anesthetics could cause permanent loss in cerebral function in

C. Scher, *Anesthesia Conversations*,
https://doi.org/10.1007/978-3-032-05354-1_52

animals. There is some literature that indicates that anesthetics could cause morphological changes in the brain and long-term impairment in animals. Geriatric patient Lenny was more frightened of the anesthetic than the surgery.

Lenny was now at an age where health issues could include postoperative delirium, aspiration, urosepsis, adverse drug reactions, pressure ulcers, malnutrition, falls, and failure to ambulate and rehabilitate. He did not consider himself to be frail and put himself through very rigorous workouts in the gym four days a week.

There is a strong bias against pain management in the elderly. Lenny's concerns were genuine. He requested a consult from the pain management service to develop a strategy for his postoperative pain from day one to day 30. He taught his residents about the evils of giving benzos and most mental health drugs to the elderly. They all move the patient from being normal to being next to normal. Lenny self-prescribed Klonopin and Seroquel years ago for panic attacks. The attacks ended years ago, and this was "never a good time" to wean them. His nurse, from her initial assessment, charted those drugs. Lenny was relieved that there would be no change in his medications.

Lenny chose Chris and Leon to be his anesthesia care team. He did not want a resident in the operating room for his case. While in the sitting position, Lenny was given 2 mg of midazolam, and an epidural at the T9 level was placed. Lenny was "hammered" from the midazolam during the epidural. The epidural was tested with a small dose of 2% lidocaine with epinephrine. The test dose was negative for both intravascular and CSF placement. The plan was to have Lenny press the button when there was pain (PCEA) during the postoperative period.

Chris planned a total intravenous anesthetic with a remifentanil/propofol and rocuronium. Lenny thought that this plan would be the least likely to cause neurodegeneration. While degeneration occurs in mice, Lenny extrapolated this data for himself. There is no evidence in humans that suggests anesthesia could cause permanent neurodegeneration in humans. The fact that there is no evidence may simply mean that you will never have evidence because it is a study that cannot be done. There are too many confounding variables in such a study.

A triple-lumen central line was placed in the right IJ, and a radial arterial line was placed for monitoring, blood samples, and pulse pressure variation. The case lasted four hours. The epidural catheter was injected, and Lenny was extubated. Blood loss was minimal, and 2.5 liters of LR were given. Lenny was transported to the Surgical Intensive Care Unit without incident. The attending anesthesiologist commented that "A good anesthetic is a good anesthetic."

Lenny slept for the first 4 h in the SICU. His delayed awakening was attributed to his response to anesthesia. While he was vibrant and strong on the outside, his brain was all of 70. Although he was sleepy, his neurological exam was normal. As he lightened up, he became agitated and restless, pulling on his drains and ostomy bag. He did not respond to nursing requests and exhibited an acute disturbed state of mind with confusion, disorientation, and hallucinations.

Lenny presented with a classic case of postoperative delirium. This form of cognitive dysfunction is self-limited and clears in days or weeks. Postoperative cognitive dysfunction is a subtle deterioration in memory, attention, and cognition that lasts a much longer period of time. (months to years). Lenny's delirium could evolve into postoperative cognitive dysfunction. The incidence is linked to age and the severity of the surgery. The incidence of this disorder affects close to 26% of patients at the immediate end of surgery, and comes down to 10% in the following three months. Of all of the numerous factors that combine to give these states of mind, anesthesia and inflammation from the surgery are major contributors to the mental health of elderly patients. There is an abundance of investigations that are well designed to give evidence for postoperative geriatric delirium.

When Lenny woke up, he was agitated and restless, pulling on his drains and ostomy bag. He did not respond to nursing requests and exhibited an acute disturbed state of mind with confusion, disorientation, and hallucinations. Since he needed to be restrained, he was given a bed in the SICU.

The current recommendation for those who develop delirium is to sedate patients with dexmedetomidine. The infusion was turned off every 12 h to determine for a neurological assessment. Most patients recover after 24–48 h. Family members are always impressed as their loved one is calm and sleeping. This treatment or any treatment does not change the course of events for the subtle onset of a long-term postoperative cognitive disorder.

Lenny went to a rehabilitation hospital for a week. His nutritional status improved that week, but his wife noticed a significant cognitive change that others could not see. While he looked willing and able to work, his wife told him that he needed more time. He was making progress, but not to where he was the "Lenny" she knew. With the tincture of time, Lenny returned to his presurgical state of mind.

Chris was aware of his ordeal. He was not convinced that he was well enough to give anesthesia in complex cases. There was a profound dilemma. Should Lenny be assigned cases that require the minimum of basic anesthesia skills?

The question comes up every day and in every anesthesia department. What do you do to an aging clinician who has a mild cognitive decline? Should Chris start to document "errors" in Lenny's cases? How does one define "error." Chris was tortured by this dilemma. If there is a bad outcome involving a 70-year-old anesthesiologist, there will be a target on his back. Lenny would not be able to defend himself. Age becomes a liability, with a pinch of bias mixed in. It was recommended by Chris to marginalize Lenny's clinical anesthesia practice while at the same time giving him projects that will support his self-worth. He made Lenny the "Director of Academics."

Lenny's career and self-worth were restored. His book proposal was accepted by two different publishers with his request to write and edit two more anesthesia subspecialty books: obstetrical and pediatric anesthesia. He applied and was awarded a NIH research grant to investigate geriatric anesthesiologists' performance and outcomes.

The dean was concerned about the significant number of geriatric physicians who were on the Trinity faculty. He asked Chris to start a database on Lenny's cases and their negative outcomes. Chris and the entire department of anesthesia did not want to be complicit in ending Lenny's career. Chris took the stand of not doing what he was asked to do. He believed that if you did nothing, the issue would go away. It did.

Suggested Reading

1. Alvis BD, Hughes CG. Physiology considerations in geriatric patients. Anesthesiol Clin. 2015;33(3):447–56. https://doi.org/10.1016/j.anclin.2015.05.003. Epub 2015 Jul 3
2. Andres TM, McGrane T, McEvoy MD, Allen BFS. Geriatric pharmacology: an update. Anesthesiol Clin. 2019;37(3):475–92. https://doi.org/10.1016/j.anclin.2019.04.007. Epub 2019 Jun 19.PMID: 31337479
3. Evered LA, Silbert BS. Postoperative cognitive dysfunction and noncardiac surgery. Anesth Analg. 2018;127(2):496–505. https://doi.org/10.1213/ANE.0000000000003514. PMID: 29889707
4. Evered L, Silbert B, Knopman DS, Scott DA, DeKosky ST, Rasmussen LS, Oh ES, Crosby G, Berger M, Eckenhoff RG. Recommendations for the nomenclature of cognitive change associated with anesthesia and surgery-2018. Nomenclature Consensus Working Group. Br J Anaesth. 2018;121(5):1005–12. https://doi.org/10.1016/j.bja.2017.11.087. Epub 2018 Jun 15.PMID: 30336844 Free
5. Katz JD. The aging anesthesiologist. Curr Opin Anaesthesiol. 2016;29(2):206–11. https://doi.org/10.1097/ACO.0000000000000299. PMID: 26705128 Review
6. Rajput K, Ng J, Zwolinski N, Chow RM. Pain management in the elderly: a narrative review. Anesthesiol Clin. 2023;41(3):671–91. https://doi.org/10.1016/j.anclin.2023.03.003. Epub 2023 Apr 28.PMID: 37516502 Review

End of Life Decisions

53

Sylvia Turner

Sylvia Turner was a member of the new generation, the growing population of those in their 90s. Many are heading on to 100. While the genetics predicted a generation of longevity, there are those in the family tree who passed in their early 60s. Improved nutrition, access to modern medical care, the understanding of the importance of exercise, medications, and a safer environment are all under investigation.

Sylvia lived alone and had no limitations on what she could do. She was independent and self-sufficient. Other than a pair of glasses and two prescriptions for hypertension, she was healthy. Family members had stopped worrying about her years ago. Sylvia turned in her car keys to her son years ago. Calling for an Uber was the mainstay of her transportation. She shopped at Citarella and hired a cleaning service who came by once a week. The "Chinese" laundry was a block away, Sylvia picked up her clothes and returned them the next day.

A significant key to her longevity was her bank account. Sylvia retired at age 70 as the Chair of the Department of Anesthesia at LSU. She grew up in New Orleans, and only some of the " lesser" programs had a pathway for women to become Chairs. Her first order of business was to have equal pay among the men and the women in the department. She was not successful. Another initiative was to diversify the faculty. The leadership of the medical school dragged their feet on that, but ultimately, they worked with Sylvia.

Between the money from her deceased husband and the wealth she accumulated from her career, she was able to pay for all of the college tuitions for her son, daughter, and five grandchildren.

Sylvia was an amazing 95 and now came the first real threat to her life. She woke up in the middle of the night with severe and unrelenting abdominal pain. She was not constipated, had not traveled outside the country, and never had a gastrointestinal problem in her life. It had been years since she had a colonoscopy. There was no visible blood in her stool.

C. Scher, *Anesthesia Conversations*,
https://doi.org/10.1007/978-3-032-05354-1_53

Sylvia did not call any family members. She was very private and did not want to disturb anyone at two in the morning. She called 911 for a nonurgent drop off to Trinity.

In the emergency room. Sylvia was examined by a surgical resident. Her "belly" was soft but diffusely tender. She had a sense of urgency and spent most of her time in the ER, "running" to the bathroom. Labs were sent, and a CT of the abdomen was ordered. Tramadol was administered for pain, which was very effective. It is not a medication that is efficacious in young patients.

The first clinical dilemma was what medication to administer for pain There are multiple physiological changes in the 95-year old that impact the choice and dosing of medications. There is a loss of body water needed to excrete medications. Liver mass is decreased, resulting in decreased blood flow that significantly affects drug metabolism. By age 80, one-half of the renal glomeruli are non-functional. Filtration slows not down to 1.l/min/year., which impacts the balance of sodium and free water. Loss of thirst adds to the problem of dosing. These changes add to the inherent bias against the elderly. Most medications that work in the brain need careful titration. Tramadol, which is too "weak" for younger patients, works well in patients in their 90s.

A CT scan revealed an apparent infection in several of the many diverticula. The gastroenterologist who consulted Sylvia in the emergency room became her primary physician on record. Due to her age, Sylvia was admitted. The plan was a trial of three antibiotics and a diet rich in calories but low in fiber.

Sylvia's abdominal pain waxed and waned from severe cramps to a continuous dull ache. Tramadol was administered as needed. By day three, Sylvia's infection turned the corner. Her pain was tolerable, but Sylvia was not taking in enough calories to make her less frail. A piece of dry toast, coffee, and nothing else. She refused to eat, and her new convoluted thought process convinced her that all foods would make her constipated.

Dr. Capella, a gastroenterologist, wanted to do a colonoscopy on Sylvia; It was an emphatic no! She knew that her paper-thin bowel with a decreased blood flow would lead to a perforation of her bowel and a clear path to her death.

A surgical consultant examined the documentation of Sylvia's case and told Sylvia that surgery was not a consideration at this time. He was not willing to inherit the high possibility that things could head south. She needed to be infection-free and in positive nitrogen balance. As the days passed, Sylvia remained resistant to eating food despite being clinically well. A nutritionist made some progress. A second surgeon was consulted, and the message was the same. He thought that Sylvia would not survive with surgery. Simply stated, there were too many confounding variables to operate.

One of Sylvia's sons, who is an anesthesiologist, wanted the surgery. Without surgery, she would die a painful death. There was hope with surgery. When anyone said that she "had a great run at 95," it made him apoplectic. The son, who knew the risks, reasoned that the surgical route is not paved for everyone her age, with pain, delirium, sepsis, and permanent loss of cognitive function.

Her son was in the "camp" who thought that everything that could be done should be tried. His mother lived for 95 years. Something in her body was protecting her. Sylvia reminded her son that two independent surgeons recommended not to have surgery. Both surgeons put an order in for a comprehensive evaluation by palliative care.

Dr. John Turner was board-certified anesthesiologist, completed a one-year fellowship in palliative care. There was some confusion between hospice and palliative care. Dr. Turner explained that palliative care is an approach that improves the quality of life of patients and their families facing the problems associated with life-threatening illness. In general, Dr. Turner was trained to relieve suffering by early identification and assessment of treatment of pain. The palliative care patients were uniformly dealing with physical, psychosocial, and spiritual loss. Unlike hospice, where the expectation of death is 6 months or less, many patients receiving palliative care are cured.

Sylvia chose palliative care at home. She actually asked for tube feedings and a trainer for her debilitated muscles.

After three days at home, her abdominal pain was back with severe diarrhea. 911 was called, and she was placed in an isolation room in the emergency room. The presumptive diagnosis was Clostridium Difficile, which was confirmed with her stool sample testing positive. Sylvia was sent to an isolation room on the ward. Tube feedings were held until her diarrhea resolved. After 10 days of vancomycin, she went back home, and tube feedings resumed. The physical activity that she was assigned to do was simply to get out and into her bed. With a bout of diverticulitis and C-Diff., she started to lose her resolve.

Sylvia was able to gain weight and get out of bed without assistance. Her aide was able to wean hers from Sylvia for short periods of time. There was life again in Sylvia, and her family thought, against all odds, she would get back to the life she had before her bout of diverticulitis.

The week of progress ended with the return of pain from the infected diverticulitis. IV antibiotics and tramadol were the same as in the first episode. Sylvia's mood slowly declined, and geriatric depression settled in.

Dr. Turner explained that depression, and not her diverticulitis, was the most significant factor that could lead to her demise. Sylvia faced persistent sadness: loss of interest and pleasure in activities she once enjoyed, changes in appetite and weight, sleep disturbances, loss of energy, difficulty with concentration, feeling of worthlessness or guilt, and thoughts of death or suicide.

To relieve her depression, Dr. Turner gave her an SSRI. This class of medications has been shown to have higher efficacy compared to any other class of antidepressants in geriatric patients. Like most antidepressants, it takes about ten days to show efficacy. In those ten days, Sylvia refused to eat, and a few days later, refused to drink. The darkness in her life persisted. She passed away after three days in a coma.

Suggested Reading

1. Tatum PE, Mills SS. Hospice and palliative care: a review. Med Clin North Am. 2020;104(3):359–73. PMID: 32312403
2. Jeuring HW, Stek ML, Huisman M, Oude Voshaar RC, Naarding P, Collard RM, van der Mast RC, Kok RM, Beekman ATF, Comijs HC. A six-year prospective study of the prognosis and predictors in patients with late-life depression. Am J Geriatr Psychiatry. 2018;26(9):985–97. https://doi.org/10.1016/j.jagp.2018.05.005. Epub 2018 May 17. PMID: 29910018
3. Cheung G, Martinez-Ruiz A, Knell R, O'Callaghan A, Guthrie DM. Factors associated with terminally ill people who want to die. J Pain Symptom Manage. 2020;60(3):539–548.e1. https://doi.org/10.1016/j.jpainsymman.2020.04.003. Epub 2020 Apr 16. PMID: 32305576

Anesthesia and Optimization of the Geriatric Patient

54

Hubert Charles

Hubert Charles was a 71-year-old anesthesiologist who trained for athletic events most of his life. He was recognized as a world-class cyclist, track coach, and participant in extreme events; the swim to Alcatraz in San Francisco and the Boston Marathon

Hubert graduated with a B.S. from Morgan State and an M.D. from the University of Kentucky. Although he chose an orthopedic residency, he migrated to anesthesiology and trained at the University of Maryland. Hubert chose not to do a fellowship. He believed he was just too old to continue training.

At 71, he was bound to a lifestyle that supported mental and physical health. His meals were meticulously managed with a nutritionist. He was in bed by 8PM and never had more than one cocktail on a Saturday night. He was well and focused and found a niche in geriatric anesthesia. He did not have a date in mind to retire. There was way too much gas in his tank.

Hubert's wife, Abby, ran track at LSU and was the mother of two girls. Hubert has been teaching his girls the value of staying disciplined with their choices to embrace excellent health. Hubert's oldest daughter played volleyball for LSU, and his youngest daughter was the pitcher on the LSU softball team.

Twenty years ago, the Charles family wanted to go home to New Orleans from Atlanta. Abby was not satisfied sitting in traffic in Atlanta and craved the culture that she grew up in. Charles chose to be on the faculty at Tulane, but could not resist when Chris made a deal that Charles could not resist.

"Charles, make your own schedule. Do whatever you think should be done to make the department better. Essentially, you are on your own. You will get the same salary and benefits that the faculty is getting."

An 82-year-old woman (Millie) is found down at the bottom of a stairwell of nine steps next to an exit of the hospital. She is unresponsive and has a bleeding laceration on the top of her skull. Hubert found her while he was making his way to the exit of the hospital after an all-nighter in the operating room. The woman was breathing comfortably and had a strong pulse. Hubert called a code, and three

C. Scher, *Anesthesia Conversations*,
https://doi.org/10.1007/978-3-032-05354-1_54

doctors and two nurses arrived at the scene with a spine board. An oxygen mask was placed, and a cervical collar was fastened.

After five minutes of being in the Emergency Department, Millie woke up. She was confused and agitated. An EKG and rhythm strip were normal. Her B12 and iron levels were significantly low enough to explain her hematocrit of 28. Her physical exam was normal except for severe pain in her right hip. An X-ray of both hips was significant for a right femoral neck fracture. Millie lacked the capacity to sign consents for surgery and anesthesia due to her concussion. A pan-CT was positive for a small amount of subarachnoid blood and the fractured hip. Hubert was paged to set up for a right hip arthroplasty.

Millie used Trinity for any of her relatively mild diagnoses. Hubert opened her medical record on EPIC and found the phone number of her daughter. While she agreed to sign consents for her mother, she served as an excellent medical historian concerning her mother's medical issues.

Her daughter estimated that the patient was 61 inches in height and weighed no more than 100 pounds. Apparently, Millie was in the emergency room last week for abdominal pain. The workup was only positive for significant fecal impaction. According to the nurse, she was a "great 82" whose brain was excellent. The fecal impaction had to be treated in the operating room as its removal would require a "light anesthetic." She recovered from the anesthetic and procedure without incident and went home. Her daughter stayed in Millie's apartment for a day.

The cause of her fall needed an investigation. Hubert calculated her "Frailty Score" based on her daughter's history. Millie was not as frail as she looked. Hubert asked the daughter about her nutritional status. As a geriatric anesthesiologist, the patient's nutritional status is important data for anesthetic outcomes.

"My mother has a cup of coffee and a piece of dry toast for breakfast.

Lunch was always a scoop of tuna salad and black coffee. One of "Amy's soups was always dinner, A bottle of Poland Springs at dinner, was her evening cocktail. This was her unwavering diet."

Since Millie's diet never changed, Hubert was able to estimate her calorie count; her protein intake and overall calorie count were not enough to maintain her muscles and bones. The workup for her fall would have to wait until her "urgent" arthroplasty and recovery were complete.

Surgery was scheduled 24 h after her fall. She was placed in traction, which reduced the excruciating pain of the fracture. Hubert wanted to "knock her out" with 20 milligrams of ketamine before they transferred from a hospital bed to a stretcher. More often than not, a patient will scream despite the ketamine. It is taught that the patient is in true pain, but the patient cannot process the pain. There is total amnesia.

An hour before the case, Hubert gathered three of his residents to discuss the anesthetic plan. This is a case where the literature is not controversial in regard to the deterioration of cognitive function after anesthesia. While it is intuitive that a spinal anesthetic and some mild sedation are better for the brain than general anesthesia, the literature is clear that there is no difference in cognitive function between regional and general anesthesia. Hubert simply did not believe the literature. He was convinced that spinal or regional anesthesia was better for the brain.

Millie was placed in the lateral position with the right hip down to get the full benefit of a hyperbaric spinal anesthetic: twelve milligrams of hyperbaric bupivacaine with ten micrograms of fentanyl.

"From years of taking care of geriatric patients, a spinal anesthetic actually sedates the patient. The brain normally receives stimulatory information balanced with inhibitory information. A spinal eliminates the stimulatory information below the level of the spinal and the balance is now in favor of the inhibitory information. The geriatric patient usually falls asleep, Sedation may not be needed. The last thing you want to do with a geriatric patient with a concussion is to sedate them. If I have to, Dexmedetomidine is my choice in the geriatric patient."

Hubert does one task at a time. The next process includes the prevention of DVTs or lethal clots in her pulmonary arterial system. Millie was given subcutaneous heparin injection, which prevented a lethal clot. There was some confusion on the orders that were given for heparin. The order was for "Heparin 5000 units SQ BID." One of the residents thought that this was the unfractionated heparin when in fact it was low molecular weight heparin (LMWH). Lovenox is an LMWH. While rare, one dose of Lovenox can cause heparin-induced thrombocytopenia. This form of heparin does not need to be monitored with clotting studies.

For patients who have a history of heparin-induced thrombocytopenia, apixaban or other 10A inhibitors can be used. These are powerful drugs, and one must determine if the risk of bleeding in postoperative surgical bleeding is more than DVT prevention.

By postoperative day two, Millie was calm, alert, and using a PCA that Hubert set up. The investigation to determine the fall was comprehensive: cardiac electrophysiology study, carotid duplex ultrasound, and PET-CT of the brain. The results of these tests were all negative. A bone scan addressed many of the concerns for future fractures. As expected, Millie had generalized osteopenia with a significant load of osteoporosis.

With a consensus from the Department of Surgery, Hubert adopted a perioperative plan targeted at the geriatric surgical patient to improve outcomes: pain, fragility, mental status, and blood transfusions.

When possible, preoperative muscle conditioning, diet, and a rigorous exam of mental health improve many positive metrics in recovery and rehabilitation:

1. Isometrics: 15 min every hour
2. Weight bearing: as soon as possible
3. Optimize nutrition with an emphasis on protein
4. Assessment: treatment of the nutrition of blood with B12, erythropoietin
5. Baseline cognitive evaluation with the Mini-Mental State Examination, which is a screening tool that evaluates various cognitive domains, such as memory
6. Calculation abilities through a series of questions and tasks, orientation, and language

The exam can be assessed in minutes by an anesthesiologist, and postoperative mental status can be assessed if a significant change arises. The Mini-Cog is a 5-min test that addresses memory.

Millie went on to live a full life. She followed every component of Hubert's plan. She was on intravenous hydromorphone for one night and then transitioned to oral narcotics. Hubert called her the day after she was discharged to make sure she was comfortable without the side effects of narcotics and to assess, over the phone Millie's cognitive function. She fully recovered.

Suggested Reading

1. Griffiths R, Babu S, Dixon P, Freeman N, Hurford D, Kelleher E, Moppett I, Ray D, Sahota O, Shields M, White S. Guideline for the management of hip fractures 2020: guideline by the Association of Anaesthetists. 2021;76(2):225–37. https://doi.org/10.1111/anae.15291. Epub 2020 Dec 2 PMID: 33289066
2. Le-Wendling L, Bihorac A, Baslanti TO, Lucas S, Sadasivan K, Wendling A, Heyman HJ, Boezaart A. Regional anesthesia as compared with general anesthesia for surgery in geriatric patients with hip fracture: does it decrease morbidly, mortality, and health care are there costs? Results of a single-centered study. Pain Med. 2012;13(7):948–56. https://doi.org/10.1111/j.1526-4637.2012.01402.x. Epub 2012 Jul 3.PMID: 22758782

Anesthesia for Liver Transplantation: Essential Critical Data Missed

55

Leonard Wallace

A 47-year-old woman, Tracey Simmons, presented for liver transplantation due to NASH and acetaminophen abuse. Two small liver lesions were biopsied, were consistent with a malignancy, and were treated with radiofrequency ablation. Initially, the lesion is surrounded by lipoidal fat. The RFA had a clear, tight target.

Tracey had most of the signs and symptoms of cirrhosis: varices, mild encephalopathy, jaundice, hepatorenal syndrome, and coagulopathy. She was symptom-free at her initial meeting with the hepatologists four months ago, which allowed her to do her Pilates and yoga. Her initial MELD score (Model for End-stage Liver Disease-) was 24. The score is based using a calculation that includes bilirubin, INR, and Creatinine. The MELD score is not the only criterion for a position on the transplant list. Pulmonary hypertension occurs in some patients on the transplant list. A low MELD score with significant pulmonary hypertension will move the patient significantly up the transplant list.

At the time of Tracey's transplant, her MELD score had risen to 34, a score that predicts death in three months without a liver transplant. At the time of her transplant, she could not walk without assistance. A transjugular intrahepatic portosystemic shunt was attempted twice. The interventional radiologist could not get a wire into the liver. Two weeks before her transplant, a temporary hemodialysis catheter was placed in the left internal jugular vein for dialysis. Her hepatorenal disease made her anuric. The plan was to dialyze her during her transplant to keep her electrolytes, particularly potassium, normal. Hepatorenal Syndrome usually resolves with a mean of 21 days.

The case was almost bloodless. A total of 2 units of PRBCs were given. All of the ABGs and hemodynamics were stable until the last hour. While the surgeons began to close with prolene sutures, Tracey's blood pressure became soft and minutes later, catastrophic to 40/20. The surgeons reopened and could find no bleeding in the abdomen, including the retroperitoneal space.

The hematocrit prior to closing was 30, and during the search for bleeding, the hematocrit fell to 16. What was not noticed, the CVP rose to 22. The anesthesia and

C. Scher, *Anesthesia Conversations*,
https://doi.org/10.1007/978-3-032-05354-1_55

surgical teams were lost. The case could be solved by first-year medical, but the emotions or the case blinded them from critical thinking. "Leonard" pushed in aliquots of epinephrine, vasopressin, and activated the norepinephrine on a pump. A liter of PRBCs was emptied into the reservoir of the rapid infuser and was transfused over a period of five minutes. There was no response to any of the medications or blood products administered to resuscitate the patient.

The EKG monitor changed from sinus tachycardia to ventricular fibrillation. Leon Wagner and Nina responded to a STAT page from the room of the liver transplantaton. They joined Leonard in the operating room within 3 min.

After cardioversion with 360 joules times two, Tracey was now asystolic. CPR was able to generate a systolic pressure of 60. "Leonard" called for a cardiac surgeon to open the chest as a last-ditch effort. Dr. Preston, an esteemed cardiac surgeon, was in the next operating room finishing a "bring back" CABG. He ran into the operating room and screamed for a sternotomy saw.

The chest was opened in less than a minute. The entire operating room was shocked. Much of the myocardium was black! The heart died. Dr. Preston, pulled off his operating gown and simply said that the case was over. Tracey was dead.

Just before closing, the attending surgeon was tying off multiple varices on the diaphragm. In the attempt to sew off the varices on the diaphragm, they went through the diaphragm and tied their knots on coronary arteries. After Tracey died, Dr. Preston noted that there were two surgical knots tied on two coronary arteries.

Leonard and the entire surgical and anesthesia teams were heartbroken. A first-year medical student would have made the diagnosis earlier. The rising CVP and the precipitous drop in blood pressure were consistent with a severe cardiac tamponade. It would have triggered a sternotomy earlier. They simply missed it. The chest could have been opened right away, and Tracey could have survived. Tracey was the first victim, and the transplant team became the second victim.

"A rising CVP and a falling systemic blood pressure is always a surgical diagnosis. A first year medical student would have figured it out.!! We assassinated her!" Everyone in the operating room would never forget this case. They passed on the next liver offered to a patient on the transplant list. They needed the time to process the event and take a few days off.

Suggested Reading

1. Tortoledo F, Izaguirre L, Trujillo MH, Tortoledo MA. Endovascular repair of accidental ligation of the right coronary artery during cardiorrhaphy for penetrating heart wound. Cardiol Rev. 2003;11(6):303–5. https://doi.org/10.1097/01.crd.0000087944.32952.1e. PMID: 14580297

The Rapid Disappearance of a Venous Air Embolism

56

Juan Rivera

Juan Rivera had prolonged grief disorder (PGD). His father passed away a year ago, and Juan could not move on with his life. He was an excellent candidate for medical school, but was so disturbed, he missed every deadline for applications. As a history major, he skimmed his books and journals. His writing talent kept him afloat to get through the year.

Juan took and needed a year off. His mother enrolled him in group therapy and a team of psychiatrists, psychologists, and social workers. His prolonged grief disorder continued to grow, and it filled his day. With medication and therapy, there was no significant improvement.

Juan knew that his father was a hero from his time in Viet Nam and at Cook County Hospital in Chicago. He had a title of Chief of Emergency Services, but remained a "grunt." Despite his title, he did four 12-h shifts a week. There was little administrative time; gunshot cases were more important than meetings concerning hospital budgets.

Dr. Roberto Rivera gave his work 110% a day. He came home from a shift exhausted and hungry, yet there was always time to spend with Juan. He asked Juan whenever he opened the front door, "who did you help today?" or "Did you work hard today? Tomorrow you will work harder!" His father was too strong to catch the disease of prolonged grief disorder. Juan was wound up differently than his father.

In his gap year, Juan's mother arranged for him to be an observer in the Cook County Emergency Room. By late September. His decision to be a doctor was sealed. Juan was ready for medical school. He was accepted to the Pritzker School of Medicine of the University of Chicago.

Juan did not want the life of Emergency Medicine that his father had. His third year clinical rotations were his time to pick and choose a career. He was captivated by anesthesiology and matched to his first choice, Trinity. The combined program of anesthesiology and a Master's in Public Health would serve his marketability better than any fellowship subspecialty. Trinity was one of the few programs that offered that opportunity.

C. Scher, *Anesthesia Conversations*,
https://doi.org/10.1007/978-3-032-05354-1_56

There are cases in a career that one can never forget. The case occurred in Juan's CA-3 year. A 42-year-old male, presented to the emergency department with severe right-side lower abdominal pain. The medical history was entirely negative. The physical exam was only significant for McBurney's sign; strongly suggestive for appendicitis. His general appearance struck Juan as a man who was in great shape. He had a passion for competing extreme events: the New York and Chicago Marathons.

An IV was placed in the emergency department, and he was forced to drink mint-flavored barium as a prerequisite for a CT scan of his appendix. In a normal patient, barium enters the lumen of the appendix. In the case of appendicitis, the lumen is swollen shut, and barium cannot enter the appendix. A CT scan was positive for appendicitis. Leon set up the operating room and consented the patient for a laparoscopic appendectomy.

The entire team in the operating room marveled over his body. After breathing oxygen through a mask for three minutes, a rapid sequence for induction with Propofol and succinylcholine was uneventful. A generic anesthetic with sevoflurane, fentanyl, and rocuronium was planned.

The ports for the laparoscope were placed as routine, and carbon dioxide was pumped into the abdominal cavity to separate the organs for the optimal visualization of the appendix. Juan was always in the moment and focused on all of the data on the anesthesia monitor. Thirty minutes into the case, the patient's blood pressure dropped to 55/23. Leon administered 400 micrograms of phenylephrine and did a checklist in his mind to determine the cause of this profound episode of hypotension. No algorithm fits for a diagnosis. Juan requested a TEE. On a four-chamber view, the heart was barely pumping. Something was very wrong. A transgastric view was in agreement with a sluggish myocardium.

"How is this possible! The patient is in incredible shape. Juan called for "Anesthesia Stat." He needed another opinion concerning what was going on.

Lauren was the first to arrive to help out. In conjunction with the cardiologists, a slot in the cardiac cath lab was ready. A propofol pump at 100 mcg/kg maintained the anesthetic. The surgeons removed the instruments from the ports but left the ports undisturbed. The entire abdomen was covered with a betadine-impregnated plastic drape.

After the intravenous contrast was injected into the 16-gauge IV, the heart started to pump vigorously, and normal vital signs were restored. The explanation by the cardiologists was that CO_2 was entrained through an open venous vessel during the appendectomy. Carbon dioxide was completely soluble in the contrast and "disappeared. The coronary arteries that were filled with CO_2 were now clean. The heart muscle normalized.

The surgeon asked Juan, if they should go back from the cath lab to the OR and finish the case. The concern at hand was that there was already a significant complication. If there were another complication, then the anesthesiologists would be in a bad liability space. An RCA would not back them. They would say to wake him up and see if his brain suffered any injury for the duration of time from being hypotensive.

Juan spoke up. “How much surgery time is there left to do.”

“I can finish the case in 15 minutes.”

“Just finish the case and get out of Dodge,” Juan was in charge here?

The plan was to go back to the OR and do an open case. “No more CO_2 insufflation!! Juan and the surgeons went back to the operating room, and the appendix was removed in 15 min. The patient was discharged 4 h after being in the recovery room and was grateful for the care he received.

Suggested Reading

1. Park EY, Kwon JY, Kim KJ. Carbon dioxide embolism during laparoscopic surgery. Yonsei Med J. 2012;53(3):459–66. https://doi.org/10.3349/ymj.2012.53.3.459. PMID: 22476987.
2. Pattni N, Arzola C, Malavade A, Varmani S, Krimus L, Friedman Z. Challenging authority and speaking up in the operating room environment: a narrative synthesis. Br J Anaesth. 2019;122(2):233–44. https://doi.org/10.1016/j.bja.2018.10.056. Epub 2018 Dec 1. PMID: 30686309

57 Epilogue: The Trinity Anesthesia Team Working Together

A 3-year-old 20-kg boy fell from a 4-foot bench. He was breathing and had a strong femoral pulse but his Glasgow Coma Score was less than 8. He was unresponsive. A head CT was significant for a 6-inch frontotemporal cranial fracture with 2 cm of brain tissue exuding from the midpoint of the fracture. A significant quantity of subarachnoid blood was beneath the brain. There were no other injuries in the patient. The mother was hysterical but had the composure to report that the child had no allergies and no medical problems.

Nina and Laurren, who were about to do a blood patch for a post epidural spinal headache, headed to slot 7 where the child was on a bloody stretcher. Nina took one look and walked over to the stock room and grabbed a 20-gauge pediatric central line kit. With one attempt, she found the right femoral vein and a wire was advanced easily up the cava. The long 20-gauge IV was all that was needed for venous access. Nina asked Leon, and James, who just arrived, for an arterial line. Leon grabbed another 20-gauge pediatric central line kit and found the left femoral artery with one stick. The wire was passed seamlessly and 20 min after the 20-gauge catheter was passed, the leg turned blue. Leon immediately removed the line and the leg "pinked up" within minutes. They made no other attempt for an arterial line. Bleeding was under control.

The scalp is highly vascular and was hemorrhaging upon arrival to the ED. The ED residents stapled the scalp to control hemodynamics. The circulating blood volume of a child this size is 70/kg and the child was significantly behind. The scalp wound was the only source of bleeding. Labs were sent from the femoral venous line for a CPC, PT-PTT, type and cross for two units. O-negative blood was released and available 10 min after the arrival in the ED. There is no significant past medical history, nor allergies.

Lucy intubated after a ketamine-double dose rocuronium rapid sequence induction. William texted Chris, who did not want to move the child before a unit of blood was transfused. They both knew that the time the patient entered the room to incision was too long without a unit of blood on board. The dura was open and intracranial hypertension was not yet a problem.

C. Scher, *Anesthesia Conversations*,
https://doi.org/10.1007/978-3-032-05354-1_57

"The child is stable. We will head up in five minutes. No worries about an A line. The staples stopped the bleeding and we can get labs from the femoral venous line". Nina was at her best when leadership was needed.

Samantha helped the residents set up for a total intravenous anesthetic. The choice of a TIVA was made if there was going to be neuromonitoring. "There is a laminated page on the anesthesia machine that has the dose of every conceivable drug administered to children. In adults we have standard dosing for Levetiracetam for craniotomies but in children dosing is based on Glasgow Coma Scores," Samantha was current with the literature that covers multiple disciplines.

"A paper came out in 2024 in Neuropediatrics. It is interesting because it has not been established that Levetiracetam is more efficacious than Dilantin, but it is growing in utilization. We are not going with mannitol. There is a strong debate going on and hypertonic saline is preferred. The brisk diuresis with mannitol causes hypovolemia and poor perfusion of the traumatic brain. We also do not hyperventilate children during our case. The consensus is, that in children, hyperventilation causes vasoconstriction and poor perfusion in the traumatic brain. Anesthetic management is clearly different in children compared to adults. Antibiotics are essential but there are multiple regimens that are almost institutional dependent. We are going with Clindamycin and Cefazolin." Samantha clearly was the self appointed leader.

Sofia came from a C-section and was ready for action. She looked at the TIVA pumps. She started many conversations with the "for fucks sake!" which is a hint that she watches "Brit Box." The TIVA should be Propofol/Dexmedetomidine and Remifentanil, and plenty of Rocuronium. I want to give 20 mg of Rocuronium every 60 min. There must be zero twitches in the entire case. We have Sugammadex! Enough said!

Ruby always had to fact check the basics of pediatric anesthesia on her phone. "Children generally require higher doses of anesthetic agents on a per-kilogram basis due to their larger volume of distribution and higher metabolic rates. The induction dose of Propofol in children aged 3–11 years is typically 2.5–3.5 mg/kg. Fuck the BIS monitor. In this case where the Propofol is set at 150 mcg/kg/minute, the BIS score will be in the low 30s. With a general anesthetic with Sevoflurane, the Bis score is around 45. A low BIS score is not associated with neurodegeneration. There is no dose of any anesthetic that has a response that matches the BIS score."

There was no consensus concerning the care of the child after surgery. The plan, moving forward, was to keep the child intubated until there was a marked improvement of mental status. He was unconscious prior to surgery and there was no reason why his mental status would be any different in the first few hours post-surgery. Dexmedetomidine was the sedation of choice if needed in the ICU. Anne, Seth, and James rounded on the patient twice a day to assist the pediatric team with sedation, ventilator management, and postoperative pain management.

The surgeons were impressed with Samantha, Sofia, and the entire anesthesia department. Chris was proud of his team. It was one of those moments in a career that will never be forgotten. He invited the whole department for drinks and dinner starting out at Pat O'briens. It was the perfect place for Chris to take a knee, pop the question, and give Sofia a diamond ring.

Suggested Reading

1. Kochanek PM, Adelson PD, Rosario BL, Hutchison J, Miller Ferguson N, Ferrazzano P, O'Brien N, Beca J, Sarnaik A, LaRovere K, Bennett TD, Deep A, Gupta D, Willyerd FA, Gao S, Wisniewski SR, Bell MJ; ADAPT Investigators. Comparison of intracranial pressure measurements before and after hypertonic saline or mannitol treatment in children with severe traumatic brain injury. JAMA Netw Open. 2022;5(3):e220891. https://doi.org/10.1001/jamanetworkopen.2022.0891.
2. Benzon HA, Butler CG, Soriano SG. Advances in pediatric neuroanesthesia practices. Best Pract Res Clin Anaesthesiol. 2024;38(2):127–34. https://doi.org/10.1016/j.bpa.2024.04.005. Epub 2024 Apr 26. PMID: 39445558.
3. Raman VT. The rise of value-based care in pediatric surgical patients: perioperative surgical home, enhanced recovery after surgery, and coordinated care models. Int Anesthesiol Clin. 2019. PMID: 31503092 Review.

Index

C. Scher, *Anesthesia Conversations*, https://doi.org/10.1007/978-3-032-05354-1

GPSR Compliance

The European Union's (EU) General Product Safety Regulation (GPSR) is a set of rules that requires consumer products to be safe and our obligations to ensure this.

If you have any concerns about our products, you can contact us on ProductSafety@springernature.com

In case Publisher is established outside the EU, the EU authorized representative is:

Springer Nature Customer Service Center GmbH
Europaplatz 3
69115 Heidelberg, Germany

Batch number: 09231155

Printed by Printforce, the Netherlands